Manning Up
In Alaska

An Astounding Tale of Overcoming
Cancer, Sailing 2600 Miles to Alaska and
Finding New Direction

Fair winds,

Dick Drechsler

Dick Drechsler

A Little Harbor Book

Library of Congress Control Number: 2009922733
ISBN: 978-0-9801512-1-3

Cover photo by Spike Webb, Radio control aerial yacht photography for hire. Email bearospace@hotmail.com

Quote from Hitchhiker's Guide to the Galaxy, by Douglas Adams, used with acknowledgment of publisher Random House, Inc.

To order extra copies of this book, contact the publisher:
Little Harbor Publishing, Inc.
1000 Main Street
Port Jefferson, NY 11777

Acknowledgements

First and foremost I have to thank my wonderful wife, Sharon. She is my best friend and had it not been for her loving support and perseverance, it is possible I wouldn't have survived the grueling cancer treatment. Her unwavering demeanor gave me the will I needed to endure. And clearly, the voyages we have shared together would never have happened if she wasn't a terrifically good sport and a steadfast trooper. She is also the kindest soul I know.

I owe special thanks to Gary Garfield, Ed.D. who took many hours of his valuable time editing my manuscript and providing me with his unique insight gleaned from many years as an educator.

Next, I have to thank my doctors, particularly Dr. Farley Yang, my lead oncologist and friend, Dr. Robert Woods, a brilliant and gifted surgeon and Dr. Alexander Dekovich from the M.D. Anderson Medical Center in Houston, who pioneered the procedure used to restore partial use of my esophagus. Dr. Gary Kiefer, my general practitioner, is the doctor I truly credit with saving my life, for it was he who discovered the cancer in my neck when I thought I had no more than a sinus infection. And I would be remiss not to thank my sister, Geraldine Mabel, who faithfully drove me to my treatments over a four month period and was there whenever I needed her.

I am blessed to have a large circle of close friends, many of whom I have known since grammar school in Studio City, California. Out of deference to privacy, I have primarily used only first names in the narrative of this book, except when discussing people whose names are already in the public domain. But all of you know who you are, as do many others. Each of you has played an invaluable part in my successful recovery and determination to find meaning in my life through the creation of the Sail Through Cancer Foundation.

Because this book deals with my fifty year sailing history, the medical, personal and professional events during the period from 2003 to 2006, and our cruising experiences between Mexico and Alaska, not everyone could be mentioned. But to all of my many friends and associates who have been so incredibly supportive, I dedicate this book to you.

As I wrote the manuscript, I realized that I have had a 25 year relationship with Catalina Yachts, now owning my fifth such boat. For the joy, pleasure and safe passages I have made aboard all of these boats, a tip of the hat to Frank Butler, President, Gerry Douglas, Designer and Engineer, Bob Nahm, Manager, Catalina Yacht Anchorage, and Byron Pfeiffer, rigger *extraordinaire*.

I also need to mention Richard Spindler, publisher of Latitude 38, who first opened my eyes to the inspirational power of my story through the article he wrote during the summer of 2007. And to Shannon Green who, after sympathetically eliciting my story, relayed it to Richard.

And to the thousands of you who have visited my website, www.voyagesoflastresort.com and either left messages in the guest book or emailed to tell me how inspired you were by my story and how much you enjoyed following along with us, I wish to acknowledge you as well. Your interest motivated me and fueled my determination as I wrote this book..

To all of you, please accept my deep, heart-felt thanks for everything each of you has done, in your own personal way, to provide me with the inspiration *I needed* to continue on in spite of the long odds.

TABLE OF CONTENTS

Prologue

On February 18, 2005, I died. Well, I obviously didn't die, because I'm writing this book, but I might as well have, or so it seemed at the time. For you see, I was diagnosed with Stage III neck and throat cancer. You've all heard the clichés "Keep your chin up," "This too shall pass," "Don't worry, modern medicine can cure anything." Not so fast, I thought to myself. This is serious.

I didn't really have time for any of it to sink in thoroughly. The day I received the diagnosis, based on a CT scan, I was told that I had four-to-six months left to live and that the cancer appeared to be advanced. This meant it was borderline Stage IV, the final, hard-to-treat stage. In a blur, I was whisked to a surgeon, a top-notch ear, nose and throat doctor in Scottsdale, Arizona, where I was living. I had first been referred to him seven years earlier for some sinus surgery that turned out very well, so at least I had a rapport with this doctor.

That same day, he performed a needle biopsy, and for some reason that still dumbfounds me, but for which I am extremely grateful, he personally took the samples to the pathologist and waited for the results. It was not good. As he described my options I made up my mind that whatever they were, I was going to stay positive and proceed ahead. But the treatment he outlined was extreme. First, I needed a radical neck dissection, during which they remove all the offending cancer. In my case I was told that as a result of the surgery I would have difficulty eating, I would have limited use of my left arm and I would have artificial veins and arteries in the left side of my neck. "What are the alternatives?" I asked. There were none. Just two days later I found myself entering an operating room, where I would be sound asleep for almost nine hours during surgery, unaware of the ravages that were being done to my neck and throat.

When I awoke I was given a glimmer of good news. Yes, the cancer was massive, it had involved forty out of forty-eight lymph nodes in my neck, my left tonsil (where it probably started) and much of my neck and throat tissue, but the surgeon thought he had gotten all of it. I was told I would have three weeks to recover from the surgery and then I would need to start a tortuous regimen of radiation and chemotherapy. Lying in my hospital bed that first night, all alone, my wife having already left for home, the fear finally began to set in. This could be the beginning of the end of my life. Luckily for me, the doctor had prescribed some very strong drugs to manage my pain, so I didn't dwell on these thoughts for long.

As I recuperated for ten days in the hospital, I resolved that I wasn't going to die from this disease, not now. I didn't know until much later just how big a step it was to adopt this positive attitude. One of my stronger traits is that when I make up my mind to do something, I tenaciously pursue my goal, letting very little get in my way. So to me, this wasn't so much a case of mind over matter, it was more just my normal way of tackling obstacles, by putting one foot in front of the other and fighting the good fight.

This book, however, is not about my struggles with the medical challenges I faced, although they were formidable, as much as it a story of inspiration. I hope that all who read this find the inner strength to forge through whatever brand of adversity life has decided to throw at you. I'm a spiritual fellow, although I'm not particularly religious in the sense of attending church every Sunday or dropping to my knees to pray. But I did know that I had a partner in my struggle, and coupled with my own resolve and the support of my loving wife, Sharon, along with a cadre of doctors and caring friends, we would make it through.

When I was sufficiently recovered from the surgery to start chemotherapy and radiation treatment, I told the doctor I had only one request, I wanted to eat a pizza. Because the treatment ahead would be so invasive to my throat, I was told that the best approach was to have a feeding tube inserted. I realized this meant I wouldn't be enjoying solid food for almost six months, so I wanted to eat something I really, really liked while I could. So with the doctor's consent, just before starting the treatments, Sharon obligingly brought home a big, cheesy pizza. I guess, in hindsight, I knew at that moment how serious my situation really was. I struggled mightily to eat that pizza, the first solid food I'd attempted since returning from the hospital. The geography of my mouth and throat was suddenly unfamiliar to me, and while I could eat, things didn't go down easily or as they had before the surgery.

But it was to be many months later when I discovered the full extent of the devastation that this insidious disease and the aggressive efforts to save me had wrought. I completed a series of radiation and chemo treatments in about four months. Allowing another three weeks or so for my throat to heal, I was finally given the green light to start on soft foods — you know, the Jell-O and mashed potato routine. Imagine my surprise when I couldn't get anything down my supposedly healing throat. Nothing! Not even a sip of water. In a panic I went to see my oncologist who was dumbfounded. So I made a beeline to the surgeon's office. After getting sufficiently numbed to endure a scope down my still somewhat raw throat, I got the amazing news that my throat was completely closed. It had literally grown shut, preventing anything from going down.

I was lucky in one regard, it hadn't impacted my ability to breathe or speak, but imagine the shock of learning that life would only continue with the restrictions of the feeding tube. I was still pretty young, 59, and very, very active. The feeding tube required that I intake sustenance five or six times a day, a process that took about forty-five minutes. So just think, between four and five hours a day, lying immobile flat on your back with tubes and funnels leading into your belly, just to eat. And the rest of my movements would be restricted by the ever-present feeding tube taped up, or more often than not, dangling under my shirt. This was clearly no way to live. I began to think my lifelong dream of cruising the world, carefree in my sailboat, was slipping away as rapidly as my ability to eat anything.

With the same resolve I summoned to endure the surgery and treatment, I made up my mind that I would find an answer. My local doctors in Scottsdale had never seen such an outcome and while they had some ideas as to how I might proceed, couldn't offer any solutions. So I struck out on my own. First I went to the Mayo Clinic. "Sorry sir, there is nothing we can do for you." Stony Brook University in New York had a surgeon, as revealed by a

Google search, who was doing some interesting throat reconstruction, but upon receiving and reviewing my files she said my case was unusual and not treatable using her methods. Same story at UCLA and several other prominent medical centers I had contacted.

By now it was September, and but for my throat, I was starting to feel normal again. It was time to pay a visit to our boat, which was some 400 miles away in Long Beach, California. At the time, Sharon and I owned a Catalina 36. There was an interesting psychological transformation occurring as well. I had always been a positive, nothing-can-stop-me kind of guy, but now, I was filled with fear of the simplest things. I dreaded the thought of driving to Long Beach on my own. But once on the road I began to experience a joy of living that I had never really experienced before. Everything was beautiful and to be appreciated – the sunrise, the open blue Arizona skies, the birds in the sky, everything. I had the top down on the expensive sports car I had purchased just before I got sick and which had been pretty much parked in the garage ever since, so I turned up the music and hit the gas. I didn't care at that moment if I got a ticket or not. Against long odds, I was alive, and one way or another I planned to live life to the fullest.

In January 2006, my oncologist called me to say that he had a former associate at the MD Anderson Cancer Center in Houston, Texas, who was aware of a gastroenterologist there who had pioneered a procedure to treat patients with my exact disability. I immediately called and talked my way into an appointment two days later. I was ready to take the next plane to Houston. I couldn't wait. Here, for the first time in over six months, there was hope. After running a battery of tests and diagnostics, the surgeon said he thought he could restore some, if not all, of my ability to eat. "Let's go," I said. It was Thursday so I said, "How about you operate tomorrow?" "Not so fast," he told me. He didn't like to operate on a Friday because in the event of complications, the hospital would not be properly staffed and he wasn't normally around either. So reluctantly, I agreed we could wait until Monday.

From Texas, I called Sharon who was back in Arizona and said that rather than me coming home, I thought she should just fly down and we'd explore Houston over the weekend. Sharon arrived on Friday and we had a great weekend, the highlight of which was exploring the Johnson Space Center, something I'd always wanted to do anyway. On Monday morning, filled with anticipation, we made our way to the hospital. It was explained to me that the procedure would require two surgeons. One, using a pediatric scope, would proceed through the canal where the feeding tube entered my stomach and up my esophagus to the obstruction, while the primary surgeon would insert a similar scope through my mouth. Over three hours, these two pioneering doctors probed with lighted scopes until they found a thin spot in the membrane that had closed my throat. Then they punctured it with a thin wire and proceeded to perform something very similar to angioplasty to open the stricture in my esophagus.

Shortly after I awoke in the recovery room, a glass of water was thrust into my hand and I was told to try to sip it. The sensation of that water trickling down my throat and hitting my stomach was probably the best feeling I had ever experienced in my life. I felt like I could bounce off the ceiling and tears of joy ran down my cheeks.

I began a year-long series of dilatations in an effort to restore my throat to normal, but it wasn't to be. On the last effort, my esophagus perforated and after five days in the hospital with nothing to eat or drink, sustained only by an intravenous of glucose-laden water, the doctor told me that he couldn't continue the dilatations and that I probably wouldn't improve any further. My esophagus was now about the size of a pencil and the tissue throughout my neck was hard as a rock, having lost all flexibility as a result of the radiation treatment. So I was limited to a liquid diet. I could only get liquids down with great difficulty, but sufficiently to survive and lead a fairly normal life without the feeding tube, which I all but ripped out myself a few weeks later. I also experienced the dream of cruising rekindling deep in my psyche. It might still be possible.

This book is a sea tale. It's neither a cruising guide nor an instructional book, but more about the things I did in my life that led me to pack up all our belongings so Sharon and I could under-

xi

take the life of cruising sailors. I'm not a particularly modest person, but I also didn't think there was anything overly remarkable about me or my story. Apparently I was wrong, because our website, www.voyagesoflastresort.com gets around 40,000 hits per month and literally hundreds of people, cancer survivors or not, have told me I am an inspiration to them. The publisher of *Latitude 38*, a well-known San Francisco-based sailing magazine, found my story compelling enough to devote space for an article about my struggles and recovery, and subsequent sailing plans.

So for all of you who have been afflicted with cancer or face some other major challenge in your life, this book is for you. I hope by the telling of my story you find inspiration, strength and the courage to tackle whatever challenges you face. A friend once told me that life is a game, and the art is how well you play it. I probably don't qualify for the Heisman Trophy, but I wasn't benched by my ordeal either and I wish the same for you. I hope you enjoy the voyage.

Chapter 1
From Racer to Cruiser

"Wake up, wake up!" I yelled to my sleeping wife, Sharon, as I tore up the floorboards to expose the bilge. Much to my shock, I discovered two feet of water and it was rising rapidly, threatening to top the batteries. If it did, it would short out our entire electrical system, including our communications. I had to locate the source of the flood and do so quickly. I was torn between thoughts of getting myself under control so I could first assess the problem, or just putting out a Mayday call and abandoning ship right then and there. Here I was, 62 years old, a cancer survivor with a serious eating disability and an only partly functional left arm, about to make a life and death decision for both my wife and me. We were six miles offshore from Crescent City at the sparsely-populated northern extremity of California, on a pitch black night, in six-foot seas with 20-to-25-knot winds blowing right on the nose, facing a seemingly unstoppable flood. Unchecked, the rising water would soon doom our nearly-new 47-foot sailboat, and perhaps the two of us as well. What manner of circumstances had led me to these dire straits?

This voyage had its roots in my childhood. Probably not too many kids can claim to have had an epiphany at the age of thirteen, but something profound was going to change my life, for that was the year that my parents decided to send me off to Catalina Island Boys Camp. In those days there were separate camps for the boys and the girls. The camps were founded in 1926 by a University of Southern California football coach.

While other thirteen-year-olds spent the summer of 1958 watching the antics of Beaver Cleaver, worrying that Lucy was going out of her way to aggravate Ricky, playing baseball, or earning Boy Scout merit badges, I was going to experience sailing for the first time. It turned out that the camp had a fleet of Snipes, a small two-man sailboat that I quickly learned to race around the buoys at Howland's Landing.

A Snipe is a class of wooden boat originally designed in 1931 by William F. "Bill" Crosby of Pelham, New York, in response to a call for small racing sailboats that could easily be trailered to events. Bill Crosby was a boat builder, as well as editor of a sailing publication, *Rudder* magazine. He came up with a well-designed, easily-built, two-person vessel with both a mainsail and a jib, designed so that it could be built at home. (In fact, the first builder of Hull #1 was a 14-year-old who built it with the help of his dad.) But the Snipe's popularity is most likely the result of the design's accessibility. Crosby published the plans for it in his magazine. So, for a few bucks, some plywood and tools, almost anybody could build a capable, durable, little sailboat. I don't know where they got them, but the camp had managed to assemble a small fleet of about six of these boats.

It was a great boat on which to learn 'the ropes.' So, while the camp had numerous activities, such as archery, marksmanship, horseback riding, arts and crafts, I quickly became obsessed with sailing. I was happy to forsake all other endeavors to be on the water, oblivious to everything but the wind miraculously pulling me along. Today, the Catalina Island Camp says in its mission statement that it provides unique opportunities for campers to develop life-long skills. Fifty years of sailing later, I'd say they fulfilled their mission in me.

Upon my return from camp that year, I was absorbed with everything sailing. I started spending my Saturdays at the old newsstand outside Thrifty Drug Store in Studio City, a suburb of Los Angeles, where I grew up. I read everything about sailing I could get my hands on during that winter. I was formulating a plan to get myself back sailing. I started saving every dime I could. I worked spare jobs to further my goal. Some of those jobs worked out, while others didn't. My friend Jack asked me if I would take over his paper route for two weeks while he went on vacation with his family. Upon his return, he got in trouble because his boss said he got more complaints in those two weeks than he usually got in as many years.

I finally landed a part-time job running a mimeograph machine in the basement of a land development office, the precursor to my real estate development career. For the benefit of readers under 50, the mimeograph machine was a stencil duplicator that pre-dated photocopying as we know it today. It was a messy contraption with purple and black ink that often produced unreadable copies. I ruined many a new shirt in that job.

That next summer, I cajoled and pleaded until my parents finally agreed, reluctantly, to send me back to Catalina Island Boys Camp. I knew a lot more about sailing by then and I was anxious to hone my skills against the older boys at the camp.

When I returned from the early summer session, my vision was clear. I had saved enough money, and during my research, I had stumbled across a kit for a Sabot that was just within my financial reach. A Sabot is a small, eight-foot, one-man sailing dinghy with a single sail and has been the sailing trainer of choice in Southern California for nearly 60 years. Armed with just enough cash and know-how, I convinced my dad to help me order the boat. He was probably dreading being asked to help, since he was not what you would call handy. Three weeks later, boxes started to arrive. I had an unfinished wooden hull, brass fittings that, to me, looked like fine jewelry, and a fresh white, crisp sail that would crown my achievement when the project was finished.

Fortunately, I already had a lot of experience with fiberglass in those days. Every summer my parents rented a house along the Old Malibu Road and I was literally living the life in Malibu Beach depicted in the *Gidget* movies that were famous in the Sixties. I had built a fiberglass skim board and had repaired numerous dings in my Hobie surfboard, collected while dodging rocks at Herb's Beach, a small surf spot used only by the locals. I had made the acquaintance of Bill, a clever fellow who had managed early retirement by buying a beachfront apartment building down the street and who seemed to spend all his time either surfing or, more likely, building, fixing and sailing Malibu outriggers. He taught me a lot about fiberglass, which can be an extremely tricky and even dangerous substance with which to work. So unlike the painted wooden hulls of the Snipes, the hull of my Sabot would be covered with blue fiberglass. Confident that I had the requisite skills, I set out to fiberglass the hull and become the proud owner of my first "yacht," at age 14.

During the process, bits of fiberglass fibers were constantly becoming ground in my clothes and skin and I remember itching for weeks. While the Sabot is easily outperformed by the more classic shape of a tapered bow, in those days, she was my pride and joy. I kept her for a number of years. Before I was old enough to drive, my father would help me load her atop the family car and drive me to Venice, along the lagoon that would become Marina del Rey a decade later. My dad wouldn't allow me to sail the Sabot out into the ocean, but I was satisfied to sail around the lagoon for hours on end. Once he was convinced that I was going to be safe, he began to deposit me in the morning and come back for me at the end of the day. So winter or summer, I spent many a Saturday or Sunday sailing my little Sabot.

When I was old enough to drive, I would, of course, push the envelope. I doubt my dad would have approved of the risks I would occasionally take. Once, I remember taking the boat down to Malibu, and disregarding the three-to-four foot surf, launching it off the beach and sailing outside the surf line in seas and winds that were larger and stronger than anything I'd encountered before. I had a pretty good scare trying to bring the boat back in through the surf. But I was getting a taste for open ocean sailing and my appetite would continue to grow.

My old mentor, Bill, and the other guys who sailed their Malibu outriggers off a gopher-infested lot near the Malibu pier, soon got wind of my keen interest in sailing. One fellow named Johnny, about five years my senior, decided to take me under his wing and show me the ropes.

The Malibu outrigger was the brainchild of an ex-Marine named Warren Seaman, who'd been stationed in Hawaii during World War II and thought he could improve on the basic design of the outrigger canoes by adding a sail. The outrigger was basically a canoe to which had been fastened a second, stabilizing hull that rode parallel with the main compartment in which the rowers sat. He built the first Malibu outrigger in his Topanga Canyon garage. The Malibu outriggers were all home-built and provided amazing

4

performance with their 192 square feet of sail area. While you don't see many of them now, the design became the rage of the beach-bum set in the late Fifties and through the Sixties.

Together, Johnny and I sailed his 16-foot home-made Malibu outrigger up and down the Santa Monica Bay shoreline. One day, in a devil-may-care moment, we decided to sail his open boat to Catalina, some 30 miles distant. We packed a lunch and some water and set out in the very light morning breezes that prevail during the summer in Southern California.

The dynamics of the wind patterns in Southern California are a function of the hot deserts to the north and east of Los Angeles. As the deserts heat during the summer days, the hot air rises, creating a vacuum that sucks in the cool ocean air, creating the moderate afternoon breezes that make this area a sailor's paradise. But on this particular day, the winds were much stronger than usual. About 10 miles offshore our boom snapped in two. It was virtually impossible to sail the boat in any direction but downwind. So at about five o'clock that evening we made a crash landing in the surf at Zuma Beach. The lifeguards there were none too happy with us since we had sailed right through a swimmers beach, but they did agree to let us use their phone to call a friend of Johnny's who would pick us up in his truck so we could get back down to the Old Malibu Road, where we both lived.

The displeasure of the lifeguards paled in comparison to the wrath of my mother, Maura, when she learned of our folly. By the time I finally dragged into the house it was pretty late and she'd been frantic. I tried to downplay the incident, but she was furious nevertheless. My mother was from Dublin, a firebrand of a woman who had red hair and a temperament befitting the legendary Irish hotheadedness. I was the oldest of three children and the only son my mother had, so I think I had an honored position as a result. But that didn't mean my mother was easy on me. To the contrary, I think she was harder on me than my sisters. She was an intellectual task master and accepted nothing but the best performance I could muster, in both my schoolwork and my personal life. My adoptive father, Hanus, was from Prague, in what was then Czechoslovakia.

5

Hanus was an easy-going sort who had a calming influence on my mother, so I could always appeal to him when the going got rough.

I think from that day forward I lost a little of my mother's trust and she was constantly worrying about what I was doing after that episode. I remember one very funny story when she stumbled across a photograph I had of a surfer riding a 30-foot wave in Hawaii. In silhouette, the guy riding that monstrous wave vaguely resembled my size and build. When I walked in I remember my mother screaming, "What have you been doing? I had no idea you were riding waves like this. You will not be doing this any more young man." She went on and on. It took me a good five minutes to calm her down and convince her that I was not the guy riding that wave and that waves don't get anywhere near that big in Southern California.

But for it all, my mother was incredibly supportive in most things. She was the inspiration for my life and constantly challenged me to do better, achieve more, be a good citizen and strive for the best. I didn't appreciate it at the time, but the lessons learned have served me well throughout my life.

Bill took me sailing as crew on his Malibu outrigger, too. If I had thought Johnny was a little reckless, I soon learned that Bill was the real daredevil. Bill was fond of waiting until the surf got really big, six feet or more, and then taking his boat up to Latigo Point where he would ride the waves. Being a surfer, I was familiar with Latigo Point. It's an unforgiving break over a rock and reef-studded shoreline with little or no sand beach. The advantage of Latigo is that when the surf is up, the waves curl from the point all the way into the cove, making for a long ride. But there is no break at all until the waves are five feet or more, so the first time I came screaming in on a beam reach aboard Bill's boat and sailed right into a giant wave, I was terrified. I couldn't let on, of course, because at fifteen, I was way too proud for that. But suffice it to say, as exhilarating as this was, I politely passed whenever Bill invited me to relive that particular experience.

And so my summers went, until I graduated from North Hollywood High School. I spent my first year of college at UCLA, where I lived in a fraternity house on campus. The summer after my first year, however, I was given a real opportunity. It was 1964, and the first production fiberglass sailboats were just appearing on the waterfront. Those early boats were expensive and to have the opportunity to sail on one was a real thrill. One of my parent's closest friends, Bill Alland, who played the part of the reporter, Thompson, in *Citizen Kane*, had done very well as a producer of B-rated horror movies, the most memorable of which was the cult classic *Creature from the Black Lagoon*, released in 1954. Bill was an avid sailor and had just purchased a Cal 25. He invited our family out for an afternoon sail in Long Beach and we all jumped at the chance. Bill intended to campaign his yacht during the local yacht club's racing season, and seeing that I had a knack for sailing during that outing, asked me to crew for him during the season. This was a dream come true. The Cal 25 was a class of boat built strictly for racing. There weren't a lot of frills on the boat, but she was pretty fast.

Because I was the junior crew member, I got the nastier jobs aboard ship. Bill raced in the cruising division because he didn't have a spinnaker and he assigned me to the job of "footing" the jib. That job consisted of scrunching up in the bow pulpit ahead of the forestay and pulling the jib through the tacks to speed the maneuver. I'm not sure I've seen anyone do this in a race before or since, but this was Bill's little quirk and since we won a lot of races, who was I to argue? I think the only skill that I really honed in this crew position, however, was holding my breath. It turns out this boat, with me on the bow as ballast, buried itself into most of the oncoming waves on the weather-beats. I was frequently submerged and more often than not, found myself sputtering for air. Somehow, I kept showing up for crew duty anyway.

During my college years I sold the little Sabot to a younger friend and didn't own a boat again for some years to come. But thanks to Bill Alland, I met a guy in his yacht club who had built a mold and a fleet of six "Dolphins," a 30-foot boat that didn't do too well in the market. As a result, the whole fleet was available for charter out of Long Beach. I always had a job and a scholarship when I was in college, so while it was a luxury, if I got friends to chip in I could usually afford to charter a Dolphin once a month. It became my practice to sail the 22 nautical miles across the San Pedro Channel that separates Catalina Island from the mainland. Catalina Island has a special place in my heart, because not only did I learn to sail there, but I also did most of my sailing to and from Catalina, which is the practice of many Southern California sailors.

Flying fish, a family of fish whose unusually large pectoral fins enable them to take short, gliding flights through air, above the surface of the water, in order to escape from predators, were a trademark of Catalina in those days. We quickly learned that by illuminating the water with the spreader lights we could simply snag them with a three-pronged hook. Sometimes they actually flew right into the cockpit. But either way, they were so abundant and easy to catch that we always landed enough for breakfast in short order. Alas, Catalina's flying fish have been nearly decimated due to net fishing and pollution, no doubt.

In those days, Catalina was a lot different than it is today. Avalon and Two Harbors (the Isthmus and Cat Harbor) had mooring buoys then, as they do now, but the cost was prohibitive for us at the time. So I would frequently bring friends along and go to Goat Harbor, where we'd anchor for the weekend. Today hundreds of boats make the passage to Catalina each weekend, but in those days, we were always alone in this anchorage. I remember those delightful star-filled nights, when I would stand an anchor watch and sit for hours, contemplating what my life was about and the other heavy subjects you tend to ponder at times like that.

I would go sailing any chance I could get. I had another friend, Gregg, who also enjoyed sailing. By now, we had graduated from college and were working, so we had a little more money. One summer weekend Gregg suggested that we rent a boat in King Harbor and sail around the Palos Verdes Peninsula, where we could treat our dates to dinner in San Pedro before sailing back. In hindsight, this was a foolish idea. It's about a 30-mile sail, which is way too much to do on a small boat during the course of one evening. We headed out of King Harbor around 4 p.m. When we got to Point Vicente, about 15 miles out, the winds picked up and the seas became very rough. Unfortunately, my date became violently seasick and swore she wanted to jump off the boat and swim ashore. By now it was dark and she surely wouldn't have survived the cold seas or a landing on the rocky shoreline. We literally had to tie her to the mast in the cabin and assign Gregg's date to keep an eye on her and try to keep her calm while Gregg and I sailed the boat back into King Harbor.

The next time we tried out the dinner-date idea, we prudently decided to sail our 25-foot chartered boat from King Harbor to Marina del Rey, just 10 miles distant and much more realistic for an evening dinner and sail. But our luck was even worse this time. After a lovely sail to Marina del Rey in light air and an enjoyable dinner at one of the colorful local restaurants, we sailed out beyond the Marina del Rey breakwater into zero-zero fog. Bareboat charters in those days had nothing more aboard with which to navigate than a basic compass. We were so inexperienced, ourselves, that we didn't even have a chart on board to plot our position. Between Marina del Rey and King Harbor there lies the Redondo Power Generating Plant. This oil-powered facility feeds its never-ending thirst by providing anchorage and underwater pipelines for an armada of oil tankers that make regular stops. If we'd bothered to read the sailing instructions, we would have known that the area is extremely hazardous, not only because of the numerous mooring buoys, but also because occasionally those submerged pipelines break loose from their anchors. They can then float, unseen, just below the surface, creating a serious hazard for small boats.

Sailing with a brisk breeze in the thick fog, with no charts or guidance beyond our magnetic compass, the only thing we had to guide us was the glow of the lights from the city. At the time, I was on bow watch, straddling the bow roller and watching for obstacles in the water ahead. With visibility dropping to less than 10 feet at times, it was a challenging job. But knowing the importance, I was being diligent. Suddenly the boat hit something and came to a shuddering stop. I raced back to the cockpit and down below to find that everyone was badly shaken, but no one was injured. Gregg and I made a thorough inspection of the bilge, afraid that whatever we'd hit had done serious damage and breached the water-tight integrity of the hull. Finding no damage, we continued on our way, only much more slowly and cautiously. When we got into King Harbor it was after 1:00 a.m. and we were all exhausted. As Gregg lived nearby, we decided we would crash at his house overnight and then come back in the morning to wash down the boat and clean up.

The next morning the four of us finished a leisurely breakfast and headed down to the docks. As we were walking down the dock we looked for the boat, but couldn't see it at all. When we got to the slip, what we did find was about four feet of the mast sticking up above the water. Apparently the boat had been damaged in such a way that while moving it didn't take on water, but as soon as we parked it and left for the night, it filled with water and eventually broke loose from its moorings, sinking to the bottom. The charter operator had not yet arrived, so we made a hasty retreat. Gregg chartered the boat in his own name and had fortunately opted for the insurance, so it didn't cost him anything, but he wasn't welcome at that charter outfit again.

In 1975, after working in Denver and taking a 2-year hiatus from sailing, I found a job back in California with one of my former bosses. I promptly moved back, renting an apartment in Malibu along the Pacific Coast Highway. That was a wonderful time. I regularly chartered a boat from the Dolphin fleet and loved the opportunities to get away for a weekend to Catalina. By then I could afford the cost of a mooring buoy in Avalon or the Isthmus, so I haunted those two venues all year long.

It was also about this time that Peter Benchley wrote the classic thriller *Jaws*. I will forever hate that book. I had two incidents within a month of seeing the movie during the summer of 1975 that would forever change my love of just jumping off the boat into the water. The first happened during a leisurely day sail in Santa Monica Bay. We were ghosting along at three or four knots, so we decided to tie a line around an old inner tube and tow people behind the boat. There were four on board, and being the skipper, I was the last to go. Once tethered 30 feet behind the boat and bobbing gently along in the two-foot swells, for some reason unbeknownst to me, I started thinking about that movie and got a premonition. I asked the crew to haul me in right away. Get this...I was only back on the boat for a moment or two when I glanced back at the inner tube and a shark swam right up to it and gave it a glancing body blow as he swam by, no doubt seeing if there was anything tasty to be had. That was a sobering moment.

But if that wasn't enough, I had another incident in Hawaii just a few weeks later. At the time, I was working for a real estate development company that was selling second home cabins and lots located in the Colorado Rockies. These mountain tracts were a real hit in Hawaii, so we registered our subdivisions for sale with the Hawaii Department of Commerce and Consumer Affairs. This required me to travel to Hawaii periodically. I always tried to wrap my trips around a weekend so I could get in some surfing at Makapu'u Beach Park. This tricky spot is on the extreme southeast tip of Oahu and is adjacent to Sea Life Park. I used to love to body surf at this challenging spot. This is a very popular beach for body surfing, but large waves and riptides can make swimming hazardous. High surf, a fierce shore break and strong undertow often occur during the winter months. The local lifeguards urge everyone to check with them regarding ocean conditions before entering the water.

On this particular trip, I was driving my rental car out to Makapu'u when I spotted a teenage boy with a body board hitching a ride. I stopped to pick him up, figuring I might get a little more local knowledge from him. During the drive, I asked him if he ever did any body surfing or board riding at Makapu'u. His response was that he wasn't allowed to surf there. When I asked him why, he replied that his parents wouldn't let him because his cousin had died surfing there. When I delicately inquired how he met this unfortunate fate, the deadpan answer was "Shark got him." Damn you Peter Benchley! Ocean swimming, diving, surfing and boogie boarding behind a slow-moving sailboat would never have the same attraction for me again.

In 1978, my boss at a small real estate development and investment firm decided he wanted to move the company to Reno, Nevada, where the tax advantages were more favorable than the heavily taxed environment in California. I was married by then, so my wife and I sold our house in Pacific Palisades and moved lock, stock and barrel to Reno. We toyed with the idea of living in Lake Tahoe and commuting to Reno, but with the money we made from the sale of our house, we could afford to buy a home in Reno and a mountain cabin in Lake Tahoe. That seemed to make more sense than trying to commute year-round, especially through winter snow storms.

We weren't in Reno long when we decided we should buy a boat. Our first boat was a 16-foot Prindle catamaran. The Prindle was a light, strong racer first designed in 1968 by Geoff Prindle. There was a local sailing club, the Sierra Yacht Club, made up of catamaran owners, mostly Hobie cats, Prindles, a Tornado or two, and one Nacra 5.2. The Hobie Cat was the most popular boat of the day and they made 14 and 16-foot versions. We opted not to buy a Hobie Cat for one basic reason. The 16-foot version is difficult, if not impossible, for a single person to right if capsized. Because I frequently liked to single-hand the boat, sailing in the dangerously cold waters of Lake Tahoe didn't lend itself to a boat that I couldn't quickly right by myself. The Tornado was a larger boat that required a two-man crew. This is a well-known catamaran because they have been continuously sailed in Olympic competition since 1976. They were expensive and too big for our needs.

One of the best short subjects about sailing that I remember was made to introduce the Hobie 18, which was just going into production at about this same time. Its designer, Hobie Alter, took three or four of those boats to Hawaii and rounded up some local sailors. He basically told them that he didn't care if he ever saw the boats or *them* again, but he wanted some of the best sailing footage ever produced. Well, he got what he asked for. Early on in the movie I was thrilled when these guys took the boats to one of the giant surf breaks on the north shore and proceeded to ride the waves, just as I had once done as a young kid spending my summers sailing Malibu outriggers. Of course these waves were huge. I thought of what my mother would say if she saw this film. She would probably accuse me of risking my life riding gigantic waves in a flimsy little catamaran.

Two of the other scenes that stand out in my memory were one where these guys invented "dagger boarding," or removing one of

12

the daggerboards used to stabilize the boats to help them point upwind to weather — riding it like a surfboard while hanging on to one of the hulls. The other memorable scene was when one of the boats sailed full speed towards the camera which was stationed on a lagoon with a big sand bar between it and the oncoming catamaran. The boat made landfall with so much speed and momentum that it sailed right up and over the sandbar and into the lagoon. That movie made quite an impression on me and I toyed for a time with the idea of buying a Hobie 18.

The only other catamaran that the local dealer in Reno carried and supported was the Prindle. He had a used 16-foot Prindle in his shop. After test sailing it, the boat and the price suited us just fine, so we bought it. The hull was a bright orange and it had a matching orange jib and an orange and yellow mainsail. There was nothing subtle about this boat, so there was nowhere to hide if you made any embarrassing mistakes on the water. It was always the standout boat in any fleet where we sailed.

After some practice, we became pretty good at sailing this boat and decided to start racing, a full-time commitment in the summer. I was 30-years old at the time and this was the first competitive sport in which I'd ever excelled. I was a low-"B", high-"C" tennis player, and while I'd played football in high school, I spent most of the time during games on the bench and only made the traveling squad for one game. That game was not a regular season game and was played against a team from a different league in central Los Angeles. I played what they called "B" football, because I was too small in high school to make the varsity team. Apparently the league these guys were in had different size requirements for their "B" team, because these guys were huge. We were badly defeated and my short appearance was so ignominious that I never again made the traveling squad. Although I was a good skier, I did not enjoy racing through the stakes. The confinement of a race course had no appeal to me, so I stuck to recreational skiing and occasionally striking off through the woods into uncharted territory, not unlike the love I would later develop for gunkholing. (Gunkholing is shallow-water sailing and anchoring in out-of-the-way places.) It's a far cry from the heat of competition.

So I was delighted to learn that I was actually a pretty good racing sailor. Today, sailors can make a good living from competitive sailing. Top racers like Paul Cayard, Russell Coutts, the America's Cup skippers and those in the after-guard positions are paid seven-figure salaries to campaign boats for a season or two. But back then, all sailing was strictly for sport. During the season I raced my Prindle with the Sierra Yacht Club, I consistently finished in second or third place. The dealer, a Prindle sailor himself, always finished first because he had access to all the expensive, high-tech sails and other go-fast options. That left me to compete against the next best sailor, and we traded places between second and third almost every weekend, with him ultimately beating me out for second place overall on the last race of the season.

This position led to one of my greater victories. Each winter, the Multi-hull Racing Association, based in San Francisco, held an invitational regatta for anyone who finished in the top three in their yacht club. This meant that the event was attended by the best catamaran sailors on the West Coast. The weekend of the race there was a big winter storm forecast to hit the Sierras, so the Reno catamaran dealer with his high-tech boat decided not to venture over the pass with a boat in tow. Unnerved, we nevertheless set off in the snowstorm. One of the other club members was a fearless, carefree guy who sailed a Nacra 5.2. This guy lived to ski, so he would drive a cement truck during the summer to support his skiing habit in the winter. But he also loved to sail and was a daring sailor who took a lot of chances, routinely winning in his class. So I asked him if he would like to crew for me in San Francisco. I was thrilled when he agreed. Between my number one rival opting not to go and landing this guy as crew, I thought I had a better than even chance of winning a trophy.

The ride across the Sierras was truly harrowing. I remember getting passed by a truck that I thought was going way too fast for the conditions and looking in the rearview mirror as he passed, only to see my Prindle, trailer and all, completely airborne and flying among the snowflakes. That slowed me down for the rest of the trip and we arrived pretty late in San Francisco. The first day of the two-day race there were horrendously strong winds. The race committee decided not to scrap the races, although they had considered it, so we took off in front of Crissy Field in 20-to-25-knot winds. We got a really lousy start and found ourselves near the back of the pack with no chance to improve our position. But as we sailed north, paralleling the Golden Gate Bridge, my crew mate noticed that there were big waves rolling in under the north end of the bridge. Since it wasn't too far out of the way, he suggested that we could take a flyer off the rhumb line and catch one of those waves. Since I had experience surfing a multi-hull boat, and having recently watched the Hobie 18 movie, I knew it could be done, so I agreed. We sailed in the direction of the big rollers and caught about a nine-foot wave, screaming past the rest of our division on the way to the first mark. By now, the winds were building and we learned later that we were sailing in a full-on gale. The course rounded Alcatraz and then proceeded on a broad reach around the Blossom Rock buoy, followed by a beat along the city front. It was so windy, that shortly after rounding Blossom Rock we lost control of the boat and capsized, turning turtle with the mast pointing straight down. But with the strong winds, the trampoline quickly caught the breeze and we righted ourselves in one smooth move, almost as fast as we'd capsized. In spite of capsizing, we still pulled out a first place in our division. The second race that day was scrubbed due to the gale force winds.

The next day, following the passage of the frontal system and with high pressure setting in, there was virtually no wind. This is common for San Francisco in the winter. The dependable afternoon breezes dissipate in the winter and unless there are storm-related winds, it's usually very calm on the bay this time of year. The entire fleet ghosted all afternoon, barely making even one knot of speed around the buoys. We weren't doing too badly, maintaining second or third place, but we were worried about whether or not we had a sufficient enough lead from the first day of racing to hang on to our first-place trophy if we finished second, or even third. As luck would have it, they finally called the race when the entire fleet exceeded the time limit, and I bagged one of my more serious, first-place trophies. And this from the same guy who had warmed the bench in my junior year playing high school football. I was excited.

The more time my wife and I spent at Lake Tahoe, the more sailors we began to meet. We made some friends at the Tahoe Yacht Club and became interested in joining. We also thought it would be fun to have a mono-hull with some overnight accommodations so we could join the cruising set. They always filled the bar on Sunday nights with stories of the great time they had while rafted with others in some of the more beautiful coves on Lake Tahoe. We made up our minds to spend the winter looking for a new boat. The catamaran dealer found a buyer for the Prindle in no time and it wasn't long before we were kicking hulls and studying what was on the market.

In the early spring we found a San Juan 24 that was in good shape. It had a spinnaker, new sails, and was race ready. We negotiated an acceptable price and took possession of the boat. We had some friends, Larry and Dottie, whom we'd met in the Sierra Yacht Club. They also formerly raced a catamaran, but had recently sold theirs as well because they had purchased an interest in a Newport 41. During the winter of 1978 -1979, I agreed to help them move the new boat from San Diego, where they took possession of it, up to San Francisco. This was my first trip of that distance along the California Coast. We had some interesting experiences along the way.

At one point early in the morning, we were shadowed by a huge, great white shark. It must have been 20-feet-long and swam parallel to us for a good 10 minutes. It seemed to be staring at us, no doubt wondering how we'd taste with a dash of lemon and a full-flavored Chardonnay. This experience forever changed my attitude towards cattle cowering in a holding pen waiting for the slaughter.

We also had an interesting encounter with a small gray whale. We were motoring along in calm winds and seas at one point when we felt a bump against the hull. Racing up on deck, we couldn't see anything in the water. A few minutes later we felt a similar bump and this time we saw it, a small gray whale rubbing itself against the hull. We have heard varying opinions as to what caused this behavior. The most likely explanation was that it was scratching itself against the hull, although one rowdy sailor would later suggest that it was really trying to mate with the boat, thinking perhaps it was a willing partner.

16

Because we were moving the boat during the only available time we had off from work, weekends, we only made it as far as Monterey on the first weekend. The weather for most of the trip had been cold and rainy and we were all pretty soaked. Because we had to get back to work on Monday, we made arrangements to leave the boat in Monterey for a week and fly back to Reno. We were a motley crew, to put a complimentary spin on it. I had all my dirty, wet clothes in a plastic garbage bag, as well as my one piece of luggage. I'll never forget the look of astonishment we got from the agent when we checked in for the flight. This was way before 9/11 and the security measures we all endure these days, but I was still required to sign a waiver for the "substandard luggage" I was checking.

The following week we flew back to Monterey to complete the trip. This time the majority owner was to be on board. I get along well with almost everyone, but for some reason I took an immediate dislike to this fellow. My instincts proved to be well founded, for he proved to be a dictatorial captain who took unnecessary risks and treated his volunteer crew like paid servants. There were no jack lines installed on the boat for the trip, so we had to clip our safety harnesses to a lifeline or whatever was close enough. He had us up on deck all night making numerous unnecessary headsail changes in large seas that were breaking over the bow. Larry and Dottie invited us sailing several times, but we only went once when we knew the majority owner wouldn't be on board.

Larry and Dottie, because they only had part-time use of their Newport 41, agreed to sign on with us to campaign our San Juan 24 that coming summer. We joined the Tahoe Yacht Club that year as well. The naming of that boat was fun. For some reason the previous owner had not named her, or maybe had removed the name to use again before selling us the boat. We never knew which, since we bought it through a broker. My wife had a difficult time remembering the name of the cunningham, used on some boats to adjust the mainsail. The cunningham is named after Briggs Cunningham, the inventor of the control. It was a running joke among our sailing friends, because my wife would call the cunningham the cucum-

17

ber. We decided to name the boat "Quecumber," something to do with being first in line and her name for the cunningham.

We had a fair racing season that year, but didn't finish in the top three. The learning curve with the spinnaker and the fluky winds of Lake Tahoe was steep. Our catamaran sailing was limited almost exclusively to an Olympic Circle course off Kings Beach along the north shore. But with our new boat, we were participating in round-the-lake courses that were far more challenging. We even learned that there is a current in Lake Tahoe. We also enjoyed the camaraderie at the Tahoe Yacht Club and were beginning to form some strong friendships among the members.

There was a large contingent of racer-cruisers among the ranks of the yacht club. More and more we were enjoying anchoring out and rafting up with the other boats in some of the beautiful, secluded coves along Lake Tahoe's west shore. The San Juan 24 had cramped quarters. There was a porta-potty, a sink with a hand-pump fed by a small water tank and a V-berth with barely enough room for two. We were spending most of the time on the boat now, almost never staying in our cabin at Agate Bay. We decided that perhaps we should consider renting out the cabin and buying a bigger, more accommodating boat. I guess like most boat owners, we were becoming the victims of what I call "five-foot-itis," the desire for a boat just five feet longer.

About this time we found out that one of the older members was selling his Catalina 30, *Illusion*, because he was getting too old to race. We went to take a look at the boat, which was moored near us at the Tahoe City Marina. We hadn't spent much time on bigger boats, other than visiting during the raft-ups and my delivery experience on the Newport 41. The prospect of full head room and a shower with hot and cold running water was enough to sell us. We promptly struck a deal, put *Quecumber* on the market and started moving our possessions to our new "home." This was the beginning of my 25+ year love affair with Catalina Yachts.

We also were fortunate enough to find a tenant for the cabin, Larry, a young fellow who was worldly beyond his years. He was an accomplished sailor and had crewed on boats all over the world. He began to open our eyes to some of the more exotic cruising grounds of the world, describing places with such unlikely names as the Dry Tortugas. Half the time I didn't believe him and it was some time later before I found out there really was such a place. Suddenly, the idea of cruising to far-off lands and warm, tropical climates was within the realm of possibility. We subscribed to *Cruising World* magazine and began dreaming the dream. I guess it was during this period I started thinking that someday I would like to chuck it all and take up full-time cruising.

Through the yacht club we met another couple preparing to do just that. They had bought a new Valiant 40 and were keeping it at Lake Tahoe while they equipped it for long-range cruising. I was filled with curiosity and engaged the owner in a dialogue about his planned trip and the commissioning process whenever I could. I remember someone telling him "not to sell the house and shoot the dog" until they knew they really would enjoy cruising. We learned a couple of years later that their cruising experience had not been a pleasant one. They moved the boat to San Francisco by truck and set sail for southern climes. Off the Coast of Nicaragua they were hijacked by modern-day pirates. The story is a harrowing tale of courage and survival. Their captors drove them 40 miles into the jungle and left them tied to a tree to die. After desperately struggling for hours, they managed to free their bonds. With only the clothes on their backs, no food or water, and only the sun to guide them, they managed to find their way back to the port where they were first taken. Having no passports or identification, they decided not to approach the authorities. Surreptitiously scoping out their circumstances, they found that their boat was still anchored where it had been left and there was no one guarding it. They decided to swim out to the boat under the cover of darkness and try to make good their escape. Luck was with them and they managed to sail out of the harbor without starting the engine or making any noise that would alert others to their presence. All of the charts and navigation equipment had been stripped from the boat, so they sailed for a full day and night until they calculated they were out of Nicaraguan waters before making landfall in El Salvador, which was a much safer country. They were lucky to find their passports where they had hidden them, so entering the country was not a problem. They ultimately sailed the boat back to San Diego where they sold it and moved on to different endeavors.

Focused on things closer to home, we anxiously awaited spring so we could take the winter covers off *Illusion*, fill the water tanks and start playing with our new yacht. We raced another season with slightly better results than the prior year in the San Juan 24, but still no trophies. We were starting to enjoy the party atmosphere of the weekend raft-ups far more than the racing, so we started spending more and more time with our fellow cruisers, enjoying our exploration of all the nooks and crannies along the less-traveled eastern shore of Lake Tahoe. I guess it was during this time that I developed my love of gunkholing.

One day towards the end of the sailing season, we were anchored near a few of our friends at a cove close to Sand Harbor on the east shore. We had all anchored off individually. It was lunch time and my wife and I had taken our dinghy over to join some friends on their boat for a meal. Shortly after we reached their boat, we heard a huge crashing sound and saw that *Illusion* had taken a full knock-down, its mast actually touching the water before gravity and the weight of the keel combined to right her. We had no idea what could possibly have happened.

Racing back in the dinghy we arrived upon a scene of incredible carnage. Two couples had been on a water-ski boat, three in the boat and one water-skiing. Apparently nobody was looking forward, because they had T-boned our boat at full speed. A woman who was riding in the bow was critically injured and had to be airlifted off the beach to a hospital in Reno. The inside of our boat was barely recognizable. They had impacted amidships on the starboard side and all the joiner work had splintered into little pieces and exploded through the cabin. Our dog, *Boca*, had been asleep under the dining table and miraculously was uninjured, although he was shaking and whimpering in fear and it took some doing to reassure him that all was well. We were stunned at the amount of damage. The hull had separated from the deck and it looked like it had been pushed in about a foot before it regained most of its original shape, leaving about an inch of daylight between the hull and the deck.

After weeks of negotiating with the insurance companies and claims adjusters, we were able to work out a suitable settlement. We had no interest in trying to salvage *Illusion*, as we doubted we'd ever have confidence in her integrity again, so we convinced the insurance company to replace her with a new Catalina 30. It wasn't too long before we were standing in the parking lot anxiously awaiting the arrival of the truck that would deliver *Kahlua* (so named because of the beige on brown color scheme of the trim) to Tahoe City. We were now the proud owners of a brand new sailboat. This was the first new boat we had ever owned and we loved the new-boat smells and the fact that we now had a blank palate on which to make our mark.

She had been pre-commissioned to meet most of our specifications, but we figured out that if we installed a heater we could extend our sailing season well beyond the usual four months that most people spent sailing on Lake Tahoe. After some investigation and pouring through parts catalogues, we finally settled on a Force 10 kerosene heater. Armed with a heated cabin, we spent every possible weekend we could on the boat. Even when it was under wraps with a winter cover we used it as a ski cabin, because our home in Agate Bay was rented out to Larry.

More and more the lure of the cruising life was getting our attention. My wife had submitted several recipes and a story to *Cruising World*, which we were avidly reading with increasing interest. One couple that we frequently boated with decided to charter a bareboat in the Caribbean. They took their 19-year old daughter with them. When they returned, full of stories about warm, tropical trade winds and rum punch, we were surprised to learn that their daughter had stayed behind. She loved the place so much that she signed on as cook on a charter boat and never came back to Reno, choosing instead to ply the warm Caribbean waters in search of adventure. She ultimately fell in love with a fellow cruiser, married and settled in San Francisco, where they started a bookstore, the Armchair Cruiser.

The more I thought about it, the more I thought my destiny might include some long-range cruising, but it seemed impossible and a long way off during those days when I spent my time

21

between the provincial worlds of Reno and Lake Tahoe. That year, we decided to join our friends and attend the boat show in Alameda. We had never been to a boat show and this large, in-the-water boat show was well-attended every year by our fellow yacht club members, all of whom apparently suffered from the same "five-foot-itis."

It was at this boat show where I learned about the tax advantages of the yacht charter business. I was prospering in the real estate and resort development industry. I could use a tax write-off that year, so we entered into serious negotiations with a Catalina dealer in the San Francisco Bay Area who also ran a yacht charter club. His name was Kirk, a fellow I remember well and the guy to whom I give credit for broadening my sailing horizons.

Kirk convinced me that with the tax advantages of rapid depreciation and the interest deduction, I could afford a much bigger boat. He also offered me a lucrative trade-in on *Kahlua*. Catalina Yachts had just introduced the Catalina 36, which would go on to become a fabulously successful boat, with several thousand being manufactured and sold. But because they had just started production and it was already October, he couldn't promise delivery before year-end. That was a deal breaker if I was to be able to take advantage of the tax incentives. So somewhat reluctantly, we settled on a Catalina 38.

We named her *Irish Mist* because of her green trim and my Irish heritage. This boat was going to be based in Point Richmond, where Kirk operated his charter company. We took delivery in Rio Vista in the Delta, probably because it was cheaper for Kirk to deliver and commission the boat there than in the Bay Area. We were on hand the day she was launched and when we saw her in the yard we were in awe of her immense size. I suffer a little bit of acrophobia, having never been all that comfortable with heights. I learned that some years earlier when I had the experience of traveling to an investment banker's office in New York City. Newly promoted, he was proud of the new office with which he had been rewarded. It had double French doors that led out to the veranda, which was really just the roof of the floor below. There was a low parapet wall around the edge. Unknowingly, I waltzed right up to the edge. The view 33 floors below gave me a sudden case of vertigo and before I knew it I had backed right across the veranda and pinned myself against the wall.

It was tough climbing on-board my new boat in dry-dock. I wasn't 33 stories up when I climbed aboard *Irish Mist*, but it seemed like a long way, nonetheless.

This boat wasn't being equipped with much, because she was going into charter service, so in a single day Kirk had all the electronics, a VHF radio and a stereo installed, and a few other personal touches we'd ordered, in place. She was ready to launch the next morning. Filled with excitement, we arrived early, champagne bottle in hand. My wife did the honors before the travel lift hoisted *Irish Mist* over the water and gently settled her into the brackish waters of the California Delta. Kirk's wife came with a gift of unbreakable acrylic wine glasses. Having just discovered these glasses at West Marine Products, she spent the entire three-day passage down the Delta to Richmond continuously and tediously pointing out how enamored she was by these new glasses. From that day forward, I have referred to acrylic wine glasses, a staple on all of my subsequent boats, as "enamored wine glasses."

As we were preparing to leave the Rio Vista Harbor, Kirk offered me the wheel. I was terrified. While only eight feet longer than *Kahlua*, boat size is proportional, and this boat seemed like an ocean liner. I told Kirk he'd better take her out of the tight quarters until I had a chance to get a feel for her in the open, unobstructed waters of the Delta. This was an enlightening little cruise, because for the first time I was introduced to tides and currents. The Catalina 38 draws seven feet, so depth became another significant factor. I remember putting in overnight at one marina that could only be entered and exited at high tide, because the entrance channel was too shallow for us to safely transit at low tide. I also remember this place because of the bees. We had orange juice on board and these bees were veracious trackers of the smell. We put in the bin boards to seal the companionway entrance. Undaunted, they would crawl through the small ventilation cracks in the boards. We ultimately had to stuff towels in each of the four vents to keep them out for good.

The cruise down the Delta and through the San Pablo Bay was relaxed and enjoyable. Kirk was an easy-going guy, very patient and nurturing, teaching me a lot I didn't know in just those three days. It was hard to leave this brand new boat after we arrived in Richmond and go back to work in Reno. During the seven years we had the boat in charter we managed to sail her a lot, however. Seven years was the magic period of time we had to keep her in charter without incurring penalties from the IRS.

One thing I realized from my brief trip with Kirk was how woefully ignorant I was about sailing. Sure, I knew the racing rules and something about systems, but I knew virtually nothing about heavy weather sailing, ocean passages, Coast Guard regulations, radio procedures, meteorology, navigation, and a host of other skills necessary to safely operate a boat in the San Francisco Bay Area and beyond. We decided that over the winter we would take the Coast Guard Auxiliary's Boating Safety Course. In those days it was a 13-week course that used Chapman's *Piloting, Seamanship and Small Boat Handling* as the text book. This was a comprehensive course and invaluable to my future sailing endeavors. To this day I keep a current copy of Chapman's stowed aboard within easy reach. One of my great loves of sailing is the challenge of this multi-disciplined pastime, although I think that navigation still remains my favorite challenge. Both my wife and I passed the course with flying colors. To this day I get a break on my insurance and a little extra pride by presenting the certificate of completion to my agent.

I love San Francisco as a sailing venue. They say that if you can sail in San Francisco Bay you can sail anywhere in the world. That may be a slight exaggeration, but San Francisco still affords some of the most challenging sailing I've experienced. The combination of winds and currents can be daunting at times and the lessons learned here gave me experience I would put to good use later in life. It's funny how you tend to remember mostly the bad experiences, rather than the good ones. One weekend we decided to sail into the South Bay and put into Pete's Harbor overnight. The worst thing that can happen to a sailor is to feel you've got to keep a schedule. Because we had to get back to Reno Sunday night for work on Monday, we were forced to depart with a forecast of near-gale force winds that would be right on our nose. The San Francisco South Bay is extremely shallow and is accessed by a narrow dredged channel. For a 38-footer, I thought the Catalina was under-powered, with only a 24 horsepower diesel engine that simply could not power us into the building winds and seas. We had to break out the sails and start a series of short tacks to make our painfully slow way up the 250-foot-wide, deep water channel. At one point we blew a tack and lost control of the jib sheet. Flailing in the wind the sheet sliced neatly through one of the plastic windows in the canvas dodger that sheltered the cockpit, allowing wind and spray to flow in unimpeded. Before we could regain control we managed to run aground at the side of the channel. This was a potentially life-threatening situation. If the boat got pushed farther and farther towards shore, it would heel over more and more and eventually be swamped by the building seas. Taking quick action, I shoved the throttle forward, gunning the engine and pivoting the boat into a tack that took us back into the deep water where we quickly recovered and continued our northward passage. To this day, I have never again ventured into the South Bay in a deep draft sailboat.

Irish Mist served me well during the time I owned her. My second trip between San Francisco and Los Angeles was in 1984 when the Olympic Games were in Los Angeles. It had been a number of years since I made my first Los Angeles to San Francisco trip on a Newport 41 and journeying down to Los Angeles to watch the Olympic sailing events seemed like a good summer trip. I was working for a resort developer in the Reno area at the time, and when I told him I wanted to take three weeks vacation, he reluctantly agreed. I assembled a rather large crew to help me sail her down the coast. The crew consisted of my assistant and her husband, another nice couple whom I originally met when they were sailing their own boat on Lake Tahoe and another friend of mine, a retired FBI agent, who was also a sailor on Lake Tahoe. Before the trip we did a weekend shakedown cruise to Half Moon Bay, about 19 miles south of the Golden Gate Bridge. Satisfied that the crew, none of whom had ever done any coastwise or open ocean sailing, could handle it, we struck out in August for the 400-mile trip.

The trip down the Coast was pretty uneventful. One thing that I didn't remember from my first trip was the pronounced change in weather when you round Point Conception, more so in the summer months when the prevailing winds are blowing from the north. Point Conception is located where the California coast makes a big bend and instead of running almost due north and south, it abruptly starts running east and west. As you round Point Conception, the prevailing flow of wind and current that comes all the way from the Gulf of Alaska is suddenly cut off by the land and within a distance of literally only a couple of hundred yards, you go from full foul weather gear to T-shirts and shorts. It really is dramatic.

Once in Southern California we moored at the Balboa Yacht Club in Newport Beach, where we scheduled a routine that allowed different guests to join us for 48-hours at a time. When new guests arrived, we took to spending one day watching the Olympic sailing events and the second day sightseeing in Catalina or back in Newport. The Olympic sailing venue was a couple of miles off the Long Beach breakwater, where the seas get pretty rough in the afternoon when the summer winds blow. In the post-Munich Olympics, the security was incredibly tight and unfortunately the distance rules established by the Coast Guard made it almost impossible to tell what was going on across the race course. More than once, Coasties with deck-mounted machine guns cautioned us to move off. That part of our experience was less than enjoyable.

Probably the most interesting experience on *Irish Mist* occurred a year later. Many of the charter users lacked adequate experience. While Kirk endeavored to train them through a mandatory certification process, it often wasn't enough. A case in point was when one of the charterers had severely overheated the engine. Kirk dutifully reported the incident to me, but thought the damage wasn't too serious and that the engine had been repaired. Confident that we wouldn't have any problems, we invited some Reno friends to join us for a weekend during which we would sail from Point Richmond to Pier 39 to enjoy some time in the city. While we were motoring out of the long channel leading to Point Richmond, the engine mysteriously overheated and ground to a halt, refusing to restart. Not wanting to spoil the trip for our friends, I elected to push on. There was plenty of wind and I figured it would be easy enough to sail into Pier 39. As we progressed, the San Francisco winds did their usual thing and built up into the high 20s. I radioed ahead to Pier 39, where we had a reservation, and advised them of our predicament. They didn't have a convenient slip to sail into, but they did have one that required us to sail on a beam reach down the entrance channel, then reverse our course and sail inside the breakwater to the outer end of the marina, finally turning upwind to the assigned slip. We dropped the mainsail and decided to perform this maneuver under jib alone. It was going well until we rounded the final turn and headed upwind towards the assigned slip, only to discover it was already occupied. We sailed a little farther and fortunately found another empty slip.

As we were doing all this maneuvering a crowd was gathering to watch these crazy sailors coming in with no engine. I hadn't noticed the crowd before docking, as I had my hands full. Only once we got safely into the slip and heard the distant sound of applause did I realize I had an audience for this performance. It was a gratifying feeling to have pulled it off with what I call good "harbor face." Unfortunately, the slip we went into was also reserved, so using a bunch of long lines strung across the fairway, we had to move the boat over about three slips and across the channel. That was annoying, but in spite of it, we all enjoyed a great weekend in the city and planned our Sunday departure to coincide with both the tides and the increasing afternoon winds.

Departing from the marina turned out to be a lot easier than sailing in. We walked the boat out of the slip and departed downwind with a considerably lighter breeze than we had experienced when we arrived the day before. In order not to be blanketed by Angel Island on our way back to Point Richmond, we opted instead to sail around the island and through Raccoon Strait. This would have been a good strategy had the wind not failed to cooperate as we approached Raccoon Strait. The wind died and with the tide change coming in about an hour, it was critical that we make it through the strait and into Point Richmond, lest we get swept out through the Golden Gate Bridge on the strong ebb tide that was forecast.

These challenging circumstances were soon compounded by the entrance of Humphrey the whale. Humphrey, a young humpback, had apparently become disoriented and ventured up through the San Francisco Bay into the brackish waters of the Delta some days earlier. No amount of coaxing would deter him from heading into increasingly fresh water, which would have been fatal. Finally, the Coast Guard assembled an armada of patrol and local law enforcement boats to literally herd Humphrey back out to sea. Unluckily for us, the timing couldn't have been worse. Fighting diminishing winds and a changing tide, we were now confronted with a radio call from the Coast Guard ordering all uninvolved boats out of Raccoon Strait so as not to impede the progress they were making with the whale. What a predicament. I couldn't get through and clear of Raccoon Strait with the light winds in time to get out of the way. If I turned around we could have ended up well outside the Golden Gate before the tide turned again, causing us all to miss our flight back to Reno. I radioed the Coast Guard and explained our predicament. No problem, they radioed back, and they obligingly sent a small inflatable boat to tow us into our slip in Richmond. How's that for service? I'm not sure they would be so accommodating in this day and age, but we were grateful for the lift at the time.

Humphrey may well be the most well-known humpback whale in the world, because he ventured into the San Francisco Bay and the Delta not once, but twice, repeating this act again five years later. On his first visit, Humphrey made it all the way up to Rio Vista, where we had taken delivery of *Irish Mist*. On his second visit he stayed closer to the San Francisco Bay and actually beached himself on a shallow bar at low tide. He had to be pulled off using a net and a heave ship. In both cases Humphrey was herded out of the Bay and into the open ocean by hundreds of volunteers who created a sound net, in which people in a flotilla of boats made unpleasant noises behind the whale by banging on steel pipes, a Japanese fishing technique known as *oikami*. Simultaneously, the attractive sounds of humpback whales preparing to feed were broadcast from a boat headed towards the open ocean.

Once back in Reno, it was time to sort out the engine difficulties with Kirk. After having the engine properly inspected by a mechanic, it was determined that the damage was far more serious that originally anticipated. There were really only two options, either buy a new engine or find someone to rebuild the existing one, at about half the cost. Kirk was trying to save money. Both the charterer and the insurance company were balking at installing a new engine, so we went with the rebuild. We spent a good four months out of service waiting for the repair to be completed. From my experience, I can tell you that rebuilding the engine was not a good idea, because it never really performed properly again after that.

My dream when I bought *Irish Mist* was to move her back to Lake Tahoe once the tax rules allowed. When the time arrived, I had the mast, boom and rigging removed at the local boatyard and loaded her on a truck bound for South Lake Tahoe. Tahoe City, on the north shore, where I had kept my other boats, couldn't handle a boat that big, so my only choice was to head to the larger, but much less convenient, south shore marina. Launching *Irish Mist* in Lake Tahoe was a triumphant moment. I had endured seven years of chartering her and now I would have her in my backyard to play with at will. However, this was not to be.

It seemed that once we moved her to Lake Tahoe, *Irish Mist* was to remain snake bitten. One thing after another happened. We had one instance where we almost lost her, altogether. One summer day we decided to sail up the east shore and find one of those deserted little coves I liked so much. About five miles up the shore we found a beautiful little spot in a rock strewn cove that had a small clear area tucked in close to the shore. It looked like it would be protected from the westerly chop, should the winds kick up. The spot was so small that we decided we'd better put out two anchors. There was no swinging room and the rocks were perilously close. As we pulled in, I deployed a stern anchor. The idea was to drive way into the cove, drop the bow anchor and then secure the boat with the stern anchor. When I got to the critical moment where my wife needed to drop the bow anchor, it turned out the anchor rode had fouled and she couldn't get the anchor deployed. I ran forward to straighten things out, but by the time she got the anchor in the water we were almost on the rocks. Forgetting momentarily about the stern anchor, I backed down hard and the engine suddenly ground to a halt, the stern anchor line hopelessly wrapped around the prop. This was one hell of a mess. About the same time the winds kicked up and because we had swung out of the lee of the adjacent point, we were getting hit with two-to-three-foot wind waves that were slapping against the transom. With all the pressure on the stern line, I started getting pretty worried about bending a strut or the prop shaft itself, or worse, the line severing and being driven onto the rocks. There was no option but to get in the cold Lake Tahoe water and see what could be done. So donning my wet suit, fins and mask, I dove in, only to find the line hopelessly wrapped around the prop. I took a knife and devised a plan. I told my first mate to pass me about 20 more feet of the stern line and then make it fast to a stern cleat. My plan was to cut the line, then quickly tie the anchor end to the slack she had passed to me so the pressure would be off the prop. As soon as I cut the line, however, the boat lurched towards the rocks. I found myself holding the ends of each line and being stretched as if I were on some Medieval rack. Since the pressure was off the prop, I asked my wife to try to start the motor and back down so I could get the line tied. Fortunately that worked. Had it not, *Irish Mist* would surely have suffered an ignoble fate on the nearby rocks.

But this was just the beginning of our troubles. Lake Tahoe was subject to periodic and sometimes severe droughts. This was to be the year of another one. We no sooner had the boat in the lake than the water level started to recede. Within less than two months, the entrance to the marina was too shallow for us to negotiate it with our deep, seven-foot draft. There was no forecast in sight for the drought to end. Faced with the prospect of keeping the boat in the harbor all summer, we elected to truck her back down to San Francisco. This would be a fateful event.

Once back in her original port in Richmond, we resumed our practice of visiting the boat once or twice a month. I had recently earned a pilot's certification and bought a Cessna single-engine airplane. With that, weather permitting, getting over the Sierras and down to the boat was an easy and fast proposition. It wasn't what

I had planned for so many years while waiting for *Irish Mist's* chartering to be completed, but it would have to suffice.

Over the next six months or so we began to notice a distinct list in *Irish Mist* and it seemed to be getting markedly worse as time went by. I asked Kirk about it and he was good enough to come down and take a look. He put a marble on the floor and when it scooted across the cabin sole, he agreed we had a problem. The boat was starting to become really sluggish to the helm. It was time to take some action. We arranged to have the boat hauled so we could inspect the hull. What we found was a severe case of blistering, where little liquid-filled blisters actually form in the outer gelcoat of the hull. While fiberglass blistering is primarily a cosmetic concern, in extreme cases it can affect a hull's structural integrity.

Thus began a saga of negotiations between me and the owner of Catalina Yachts. He at first suggested that we sail the boat down to his yard in Oxnard where he would repair the damage at cost. I told him that I didn't think the hull was seaworthy and that I wasn't about to risk my life or anyone else's to move the boat by sea. We finally agreed to hire a surveyor to inspect the boat and make a report by which we would both be bound. When he arrived, the surveyor's initial comment was that he had never seen such a serious case of blistering. He was actually able to stick his finger right through the outer hull and into the core. This was a much more serious situation than I had envisioned.

I said earlier I had a 25-year love affair with Catalina Yachts. I had never met or dealt with the owner before, and although he could be brusque and gruff on the surface, he is a remarkable man and as honest and honorable as they come. Upon receiving the surveyor's report, he agreed to take the boat as a trade-in on a new boat, giving me fair market value. He arranged to sell me a new boat at cost through a local dealer in the Bay Area. This deal worked out incredibly well for me. As I recall, I actually owed $13,000 less than the cost of the new boat after the trade-in, so I put a nice hunk of cash in the bank. I also achieved another goal. I was able to convince Catalina Yachts to trade my 38 for a Catalina 36, the boat I had wanted in the first place. The deal was sealed and we even learned that a new Catalina 36 was immediately available in the Bay Area.

To this day we do not know what caused the severe blistering on our Catalina 38. There are two theories. In 1983, the year it was built, the government had forced all yacht manufacturers to change the mixture they used for the fiberglass in order to be more environmentally friendly. Faced with the challenge, all of the boat manufacturers began experimenting with different blends and blistering became a problem for many years to come. The builder also surmised that the problem might have been related to moving the boat from salt water to fresh water and then back again so fast. I personally never ascribed much to that theory. But the bottom line to the whole story was that Catalina Yachts made good on their product and I was about to take delivery of another new yacht, my fourth Catalina in a decade.

Chapter 2
New Yacht, New Life

There was a very popular television show in the late Eighties called *L.A. Law*. It was centered around a Los Angeles law firm that took on controversial cases. Two of the characters, played by Jill Eikenberry and Michael Tucker, who were husband and wife in real life, were a couple of single lawyers. Michael Tucker's character, the *schlumpy* Stuart Markowitz, had been trying for months to strike up a relationship with Jill Eikenberry's character, Ann Kelsey. In one episode that was particularly memorable, Markowitz was lamenting that he was getting nowhere with Kelsey and that if things didn't change fast, their next date would probably be their last. He learns of the "Venus Butterfly," which would apparently make him irresistible, from a client he's representing in his role as a defense attorney. We never knew the specifics, but the next morning after the date, Kelsey was head over heels for Markowitz and the two characters went on to get married in the show. From then on I used to kid around with my friends that I had no idea what it was, but I wanted one!

So when it came time to name the new boat, it seemed to me that "Venus Butterfly" would be a perfect name. It had this TV connotation as some kind of an aphrodisiac and yet, it also had a lyrical beauty that conjured up images of butterflies floating in space. It seemed perfect. My wife was a little more skeptical. She didn't know what it meant either, but as we now had a young daughter she didn't think that even the hint of an aphrodisiac connection was appropriate. I convinced her it would be fine and we ultimately named the boat *Venus Butterfly*.

By the time we took delivery of the new Catalina 36, our lifestyle had changed significantly. For one thing, we had taken advantage of another tax program and purchased a second boat, which we based in the Caribbean. In response to the coup in Granada and the take-over by the communist forces within the country, President Reagan had responded by sending in U.S. troops to recapture the island nation and re-install the duly elected democratic government. Because the root causes of the problems were economic blight and poverty, President Reagan adopted his Caribbean Basin Initiative. This program of military and economic assistance, effectively extended to U.S. citizens all of the current investment tax incentives, including capital gains and accelerated depreciation, to investments made in the certain select countries of the Caribbean. This made it possible to purchase a charter boat in the Caribbean and get the same tax advantages I had when I first put *Irish Mist* into the charter business.

Second, I had recently achieved a degree of success in the advertising business, primarily through one single promotion. My partner and I had gained the rights to use Continental Airlines' name on a direct mail piece offering a free companion airline ticket as an incentive for attending a resort promotion. The advertising campaign was wildly successful and we were paid a royalty for each piece of outgoing mail displaying the Continental Airlines logo. There was an interesting twist to this story. The response was actually too good. The program was costing our client a lot more than originally budgeted, as he had to pay for that second ticket when it was used. At about the same time, Continental Airlines experienced a labor strike and flights were suspended for several months. During the strike, the expiration date on the offer passed. We weren't happy that people didn't get their vacations, but it was beyond our control and the strike did work to our client's economic advantage.

There were hundreds of complaints filed with the California Attorney General's office and they initiated an investigation of the whole promotion. As it was clearly beyond our control, no action was taken by the Attorney General. But apparently they leaned on Continental Airlines, because the airline unilaterally agreed to extend the deadline. Our client refused to pay for flights redeemed after the original deadline on the basis that he did not agree to extend that deadline. Unfortunately, that was the end of both the promotion and the client, but over the one-year period during which we conducted the campaign, we did quite well.

My partner in the advertising agency, Jerry, was familiar with a charter company in the Caribbean called the Moorings. They are extremely well established now, but they weren't so well known on the West Coast back then. He suggested that with the new tax treatment of Caribbean investments, maybe we should each buy a charter yacht to take advantage of the new rules. It sounded like a good idea. So, sight unseen, we each signed a contract to purchase a new Beneteau (Moorings) 51 to be placed in charter service in St. Lucia in the West Indies.

During the pendency of the transaction we flew down to Tortola, the largest island in the British Virgin Islands, so we could sea-trial an identical Beneteau 51 to make sure we liked the boat before we closed the deal. It was a fantastic boat and this being my first Caribbean experience, I was thrilled. Since most of the money to buy this boat had come from our advertising agency, we decided to name our Beneteau *Ad Ease*. Jerry named his *Residual Fun*. Jerry, our wives and I had a great time during this period and would usually buddy-boat and travel together. As for my wife and I, we would own our boat and keep it in charter for six years. During this time we tried to make two or three trips a year to the Caribbean to explore different islands and cultures.

The guidebooks all say that when you pack for a winter trip to the Caribbean you need to ignore the weather outside and leave all your jackets, sweaters and warm clothes at home. With snow on the ground in the Sierras and occasional snow in Reno proper, I just couldn't believe it. So, of course, I was over-packed on this first trip. I learned better and on future trips limited my wardrobe to a few pairs of shorts and T-shirts, two bathing suits, one pair of long pants, and a sports shirt for more formal evenings.

My years sailing the Caribbean were packed with discovery and adventure, as well as some tremendously amusing experiences. The funniest experience related to my stepdaughter during our first trip to St. Lucia to see the new boat. The routine was to arrive on the first day and spend that night in the local hotel in Marigot Bay. The following morning was consumed with a skipper's chart briefing, a boat check-out and provisioning food and supplies for the full two weeks of the sailing vacation. Just as we were loading the frozen food aboard to be stowed in the freezer, before it could thaw in the hot tropical sun, my wife told me that her daughter had started her first menstrual cycle. My wife asked if I would tend to getting what she needed so she could keep up with the stowage of provisions before the food spoiled. Obligingly, I left my stepdaughter and wife to attend to the pantry while I marched up to the customer service office. I discreetly inquired of the woman behind the desk if she could direct me to a store where I might find the appropriate supplies. To this day I still laugh out loud at her response. With one eyebrow raised and in a clearly disapproving tone, she looked down her nose at me and loftily asked "Does this child not have a mother?" For many years after that, whenever my daughters would act up, I would jokingly ask my wife, "Does this child not have a mother?"

While that first trip was exciting, it was also a humbling experience. It turns out that charter boats in the Caribbean are often scorned by local cruising yachts. We were sure we had bought a huge, dream yacht with the purchase of *Ad Ease*, but when we arrived in Marigot Bay, we were chagrined to find that we were one of the smallest boats in the harbor. Most of the people on the larger cruising yachts wanted nothing to do with us, although the crew on one of the sailing mega-yachts docked across from us at one point did warm up when they found out we actually owned the boat. I remember being intrigued back in those days by the presence of white domes on many of the larger cruising boats, so I asked a member of this crew what the dome on their boat was. He replied it was a "BRT." Having no idea what that was, and not particularly interested in showing off my ignorance, I nodded knowingly and let it pass. I wondered all night long what the hell a BRT might be, so I revisited the issue the next morning and the fellow laughingly replied, "Oh, that's a Big Round Thing." Now I really felt too stupid to pursue the subject further, so I laughed and left no wiser than when I'd first inquired. It would be many years before I found out that a BRT was really a dome to house various gyro-stabilized satellite communication receivers.

Once provisioned, if sailing south towards Bequia, Union Island, the Tobago Keys or the Grenadines, the usual plan was to leave around noon and sail down-island to a little town on the southwest corner of St. Lucia in the West Indies called Soufrière. Soufrière was a sleepy little fishing village that had actually been the capital of St. Lucia during French rule, but had fallen on poorer times when the capital was moved to Castries. Over the years we made friends with many of the young boys of the town. The Moorings in St. Lucia had a custom of sending each boat out with a big branch of fresh bananas tied to the stern rail for consumption as they ripened during the voyage. The first time we arrived in Soufrière we were greeted by a half dozen boys who swam out to meet us, volunteering to check our anchor with a dive mask for a nickel and to watch the boat while we went ashore or explored the nearby attractions by dinghy. They were great kids, and we grew particularly close to two of them, Bernard and his brother Franklin.

Bernard was about twelve when we first met him and Franklin maybe five years younger. They were such innocent boys in those days. Soufrière, being at the southern tip of St. Lucia, was pretty isolated. Most of its contact with the outside world was with visiting yachtsmen such as us. The young kids wore loin cloths and spent their days playing on the beaches of paradise.

It usually was frowned upon by our fellow yachtsmen and charterers to allow the local kids below decks. We pretty much adhered to this rule. Although we would leave them alone on board with the cabin locked up to watch over things above decks for a nickel, in reality it was just a way to give them a nickel, since all the kids were well-behaved and we weren't aware of any theft or other problems.

But one year, for Bernard, I made an exception. Bernard had ambitions to go to college in the United States. He was a bright kid with an inquiring mind and I had developed a real fondness for him. He worked for several hours after school each day in the local ice cream store for fifteen cents a day. Most of those kids, at first anyway, had little knowledge of the outside world. That would change later. One day Bernard asked if he could see the engine, so this is when I made the exception and took him below to have a look. His face betrayed incredulity at seeing the interior of the boat for the first time.

Bernard understood that the boat was in charter and had seen it with other people on board. He asked, a little sheepishly, if I would tell him how much people had to pay to charter *Ad Ease*. When I told him, I could see the wheels turning. Pretty soon he got a big smile on his face and said that if he made that much money he could retire before he turned 21-years old. I waited for a moment and when the light didn't dawn, I told him he was forgetting something. "Bernard, where are you going to get a boat?" He thought for a minute and then asked me how much a boat like this would cost. When I told him, poor Bernard was deflated. His plan to retire at 19 or 20 evaporated before his eyes.

Were I a sociologist, it would have been fascinating, and tragic, to watch and document what happened to that little town. About three years after I started visiting on a regular basis, the town installed a satellite dish to bring U.S. television feeds to the residents. In those days CNN was just coming into its own. Dallas was the reigning TV series, and like today, local news feeds were full of stories of violent crimes. In just one year of exposure to American television, things changed dramatically. The kids didn't want a nickel to watch the boat anymore, they wanted a buck. And there was good reason, because some of the older kids had taken to petty theft. That year, we had the entire bunch of bananas stolen from the stern rail. We had left Franklin, Bernard's kid brother, alone to watch the boat. When we returned he said he had been threatened and overpowered by a group of older boys. Suddenly their little paradise in this faraway corner of the world wasn't good enough. They all wanted to go to the United States. They had little appreciation of the need for education or hard work, thinking instead that if they could get to the United States they would automatically have it made.

There were still touching moments and experiences I'll never forget. At some point Bernard expressed his desire that we meet his parents and proudly told us that his mother wanted us to come to dinner. We had done what we could for Bernard and his brother over the years, without trying to make it look like charity. He explained that his mother wanted to repay our kindness. We were honored. We took as much food and drink as we thought we could get away with and still not look patronizing. Bernard's parents were lovely, simple, honest and hard-working people. They were

38

very modest and shy and continuously tried to apologize for the quality of their home. We would hear none of it and once the ice was broken, we had a wonderful, laughter-filled evening. It was a great experience for all of us. Bernard was really proud and pleased that we had all gotten along so well.

It has been many years now since I visited Soufrière. It will be interesting, indeed, to return some day on a future voyage and find out how Bernard and his family have fared over the years. I often wonder if Bernard made it to college in the States.

The town of Soufrière is well known from pictures of its landmark, the Pitons, two volcanic "plugs" that frame the town. A volcanic plug, also called a volcanic neck or lava neck, is a volcanic landform created when magma hardens within a vent on an active volcano. When forming, a plug can cause an extreme build-up of pressure if volatile-charged magma is trapped beneath it, and this can sometimes lead to an explosive eruption. If a plug is preserved, erosion may remove the surrounding rock while the erosion-resistant plug remains, producing a distinctive landform. These landmarks rise directly up from the coral reef beds and form part of a UNESCO World Heritage Site. The region is popular for snorkeling and scuba diving.

Although the exact location is disputed by historians, the town is also reputed to be the birthplace of Napoleon's Empress Joséphine de Beauharnais, whom it is certain, spent much of her childhood in the town on her father's plantation.

Sailing in the Caribbean was a real dream, although I can't say I liked everything about it. On one trip, we decided to visit Martinique, which is officially designated as an "overseas department" of France and part of the Republic. The main town is Fort-de-France. I'm not sure about now, but in those days the town had an open sewer system that ran adjacent to all the streets and was unsightly and odorous. This was compounded by the fact that the locals used the sewer channels as public, outdoor restrooms. I'm not particularly modest, but this practice did not appeal to me.

Entering the Moorings ownership and lease-back program in those days had another great benefit. As the Moorings continued to grow, they decided to add additional bases around the world.

Owners now had the ability to exchange for a sister-ship in another venue. I had always dreamed of sailing in the South Pacific one day. I once arranged a crewed charter in Hawaii to try to get a taste of South Pacific sailing, but unfortunately when we arrived to embark on our trip, the weather had turned foul with gale force winds and high seas forecast between the islands. The captain that ran the charters canceled it on the spot, leaving us to scurry around and secure a hotel room at the last minute. It was particularly annoying that he made us pay for the food, despite our not having a refrigerator large enough to hold 10 days of food back in a Honolulu hotel room.

When the Moorings opened a base in Tahiti, Jerry and I couldn't wait to take a sailing vacation there. The Moorings base was in Raiatea, in Tahiti's leeward island group, which consists of Raiatea, Huahine, Tahaa and Bora Bora. We planned a two-week trip and invited another couple to join us. My partner and his wife invited his sister-in-law and her husband along on their boat, so we were a group of ten on two boats, counting our two children.

Tahiti truly fits the soothing images conjured up in James Michener's *Return to Paradise* of idyllic, lush green islands surrounded by barrier reefs that protect the islands from the sea. Tropical cyclones, like hurricanes in the Atlantic and Caribbean Sea, are a serious concern during the months of November through April. While we had pushed the envelope by traveling to the Caribbean many times towards the onset of the hurricane season, we didn't want to take any such chances with our trip to Tahiti.

The chart briefing in Tahiti is a bit different than that given in the Caribbean bases. To begin with, one of the first things you learn is that there are a lot of things in the South Pacific waters that can kill you. We were warned that some sea snakes can be aggressive. Scorpion fish, which sit on the sand in shallow tide pools, are well camouflaged and have a dangerous sting. What really got our attention was the description of the cone snail. They have a poison gland containing neurotoxins that is launched out of their mouths in a harpoon-like action that they use for stunning and killing fish and invertebrates. They too are found in shallow tidal pools where they bury themselves in the sand with only their stinger protrud-

40

ing. As it was explained to us, if you get stung by a larger one of these, say your prayers, because you've only got about fifteen minutes to live. I don't know if this was an exaggeration or not, but suffice it to say whenever we waded through shallow tidal pools to get to a beach, we wore reef shoes and kept a keen eye on the sand ahead of us at each step.

The other big concerns are the coral heads that dot the waters inside the coral reefs and are a hazard to navigation. These often can't be spotted unless the sun is directly overhead or nearly so. For this reason, it is recommended that arrivals and departures from these spectacular lagoons be planned for midday and that an attentive bow lookout be maintained. We found this to be particularly useful information on our visits to Huahine and Bora Bora.

Other than those warnings, sailing in the South Pacific was pretty straightforward. On the passages between islands you can encounter some large seas and we did have more than one incidence of long-period sea swells of 10 feet or more. Wherever there is freshwater runoff from an island, such as near the mouth of a river, the coral does not grow. This leads to natural openings in the barrier reefs forming convenient channels to enter these protected harbors. But as silt collects in these openings, they can be shallower than the surrounding waters, causing the seas to heap up over the resulting bars. We experienced these conditions when we arrived at Huahine. We watched a freighter enter ahead of us and it really got our attention when this 100-plus foot ship would disappear between the steep swells. We held our breath as we made our own entry to the lagoon.

Huahine was my personal favorite. When we arrived there, we sailed through the Avamoa Pass at the town of Fare, which we bypassed altogether. Instead, bow lookouts in place, we worked our way down the inside of the barrier reef as far as one could go, about 18 miles. In those days, there was only a small bed and breakfast there and the entire end of the lagoon was a marine sanctuary. I could have easily stayed and lived there happily ever after. Each morning a truck would come by with fresh baguettes. Much as we have a mailbox in front of our homes, the homes in Huahine also had baguette boxes in which the driver would deposit a fresh

41

baguette each day. I learned about this our first day there, so each morning I would dinghy in early enough to intercept the truck and purchase that day's supply of baguettes for the two boats. In the afternoons, we got in the habit of going ashore to the bed and breakfast where we'd have glacé (the local name for ice cream) and a beer or two. It was idyllic. I hated to leave, but we had much to see in Tahaa and Bora Bora.

I do have a good fish story from this trip. My partner and his brother-in-law, who was traveling with them, were both avid fisherman. *En route* to Tahaa they were about a half-mile astern. One minute they were sailing along smoothly behind us. The next thing we knew, they were headed up into the wind, their crew struggling to lower the violently flogging sails. Once it looked like the situation was under control I radioed over and asked what was going on. They responded that they had a marlin on the line and that they had to head up suddenly to slow the boat before they snapped the line. Figuring it could take several hours to land a marlin, I told them we'd sail on and meet them when they finally reached port later in the day.

Almost four hours after we arrived in port, they sailed in and anchored nearby. I hopped in the dinghy and went over to see if they had caught the marlin when they proudly showed me the 30-pound tuna they had landed. I started laughing out loud and asked them what they had been smoking when they told me they'd hooked a marlin. They all swore they had seen a marlin on the line and were at a loss to explain it. When they started to clean the tuna, however, we found three holes right through it. Apparently, they had hooked the tuna in the first place, but a marlin had repeatedly speared it. What they saw was the marlin jumping out of the water with the speared tuna, but at the distance and speed with which it all happened, they didn't know what was actually taking place until we discovered the spear holes in the tuna. Talk about the one that got away!

Jerry had the extreme misfortune of contracting dengue fever shortly after we arrived in Tahaa. Dengue fever usually starts with a sudden onset of severe headache, muscle and joint pain, fever and rash. Severe pain gives it the name *break-bone fever* or *bone-crusher disease*. He was in utter agony. We had no idea what was wrong, so I volunteered to take my dinghy the three miles to the nearest town and see if I could find a doctor. Fortunately, the doctor made house calls and although he had never seen any patients on a yacht before, he was good humored about it and accompanied me back in the dinghy to tend to my partner. Dengue fever is spread by mosquitoes, so he must have contracted it while we were in Huahine.

Although Jerry had an inexperienced crew, they felt they had learned enough that they could cut their trip short and get the boat back to Raiatea. There they would find better medical facilities for Jerry and get him additional treatment, if necessary. Reluctantly, we bid them farewell as they insisted we continue on without them. They left the next morning while we stayed another day or two, awaiting word that they'd arrived safely, before heading on to Bora Bora.

I had drooled over scenic pictures of Bora Bora in the cruising magazines over the years, particularly the distinctive hotel rooms with thatched roofs that are commonly built on pilings over the water with individual piers leading to them. I had always wanted to see that first hand and Bora Bora did not disappoint. The enduring memory of Bora Bora was the color of the water inside the lagoons. You can't do justice to the bright emerald green and azure blue waters, even with the best of cameras and lighting. The colors of these waters simply have to be seen to be fully appreciated.

We were able to keep in touch with my partner's boat using the VHF radio, and we knew that while they had safely made it back to Raiatea, he was very ill and all aboard were worried. The Moorings managed to arrange for another doctor to visit the boat, and once the diagnosis was confirmed, there wasn't anything else anybody could do but just wait it out. His illness and the need to cut short their voyage put a damper on the rest of our trip as well. I was glad when we decided to go back to Raiatea a couple of days early so I could be there to help out and coordinate any further medical treatment that might be required. Fortunately, by the time we returned, the fever had broken and within 48 hours my partner had made an almost complete recovery.

From the Moorings' base in Raiatea we flew back to Papeete, where we planned to spend a couple of days before flying back home. This is where I got the real shock of the trip. We had been subsisting primarily on the provisions packed aboard before we sailed out of Raiatea and the fish we caught along the way, so we hadn't experienced the expenses of food and lodging in the cosmopolitan city of Papeete. We were stunned at the prices. There were no sales or VAT taxes in Tahiti, except on hotel accommodations, but the prices for everything were exorbitant. Apparently the government eased the burden on the locals with an annual subsidy, but no such break was available for tourists. One day we stopped along the shore for a quick lunch at a local roadside stand. Lunch, which consisted of four hamburgers with fries and four Cokes, was $136.00 U.S. This was in the mid-Eighties. Understandably, I was extremely relieved when we boarded our plane for home.

Back home, my world was to change dramatically. In 1988, Robert ("Bob") Beaumont, my employer and mentor for almost two decades, died suddenly at the young age of 48. When Bob died his Estate was governed by three trustees, all of whom had been employees or consultants to the company, including Bob's lawyer and accountant. Without Bob's presence, and because so much of my life revolved around sailing, I saw no reason to stay in Nevada for long. Within a couple of years of Bob's death I had organized things sufficiently that the company didn't really need my services any longer. By now I was getting homesick for Southern California and I had begun putting out feelers looking for a job back there. I remember getting a call right before Christmas and being offered a job with the stipulation that I must start before January 2. This was impossibly short notice given that I had a family with young daughters in school. I flew down to Laguna Hills, in Orange County, California and successfully negotiated an attractive employment package. Immediately after Christmas I started to make hurried arrangements. Logistically, one challenge was to move the boat. Also, I reasoned I could save a lot of money by living temporarily aboard while we found a house in Orange County, sold the one in Reno and resettled the family. The move was further complicated by the fact that my wife really did not want to move. She was comfortable in Reno and didn't care to relocate to Southern California. However, at this point we really didn't have much choice. My job with Beaumont's company was over and there were no appropriate opportunities for me in Reno. There was little I could do, other than to take a deep breath and move forward. With little time to lose, I hurriedly arranged to have a Loran navigation system and an autopilot installed on *Venus Butterfly* for the trip south from San Francisco.

Finding crew to help me move the boat to Los Angeles over the holidays wasn't easy, but I did know the fellow I'd been paying for several years to look after my boat and do occasional work on it, who volunteered to help me out. He was a fascinating guy who had once crewed on the Whitbread Round the World Race (now known as the Volvo Ocean Race). I was in awe of anyone with the courage and endurance to have participated in this race, especially in the early days when the technology and safety-equipment weren't nearly as sophisticated as now.

My friend's descriptions of his passage through the Southern Ocean were particularly riveting and made the long hours of our own voyage pass quickly. He described the Southern Ocean as a place where icicles are a permanent fixture on the lifelines, winds blow steadily at gale and often greater force, and the sea swells are higher than the mast, with 10-to-20-foot whitecaps breaking off their tops. He said that the whitecaps weren't a problem during the day because you could see them cresting in time to maneuver to safety as you emerged from the darkness of the deep troughs, but at night, with the wind roaring, you only had your sense of hearing to rely on and the direction of the sounds was deceiving. I remember commenting that I might find that interesting if I could be airlifted by helicopter and spend one day aboard in those conditions, silently vowing never to include the Southern Ocean in my future cruising plans.

We set sail together a few days after Christmas under clear, cool skies and favorable winds. He had agreed to go as far as Santa Barbara where he would jump ship and fly back to San Francisco. I had arranged for one of my oldest friends, Fred, and his wife Suzi, to meet me in Santa Barbara and help me crew the boat for the rest of the trip to Oceanside. We had a great time, celebrating New Years Eve in Marina del Rey before pushing on.

I found myself without family and experiencing live-aboard status for the first time. Part of the deal I made with my new employer was that I could fly home every Friday afternoon for the first 90 days until we got settled into a new home in the area. Being from Los Angeles, I didn't know many people in Orange County. This was a lonely time for me, but I was really happy to be back in Southern California and planned to move the boat up to Los Angeles permanently once the family was settled. In the meantime, my new boss took pity on me and after a couple of weeks of my living on the boat, he moved me into a condominium project that he managed near the office. I actually liked living on the boat, but it was a long drive from Oceanside to Laguna Hills, and I didn't much care for that, so I was happy to make the move.

Unfortunately, my plan to move the boat to the Los Angeles area didn't pan out at first. Slips in those days were at a premium. Although I had my name on waiting lists at a number of marinas, nothing was opening up. At the same time Oceanside had a maximum of 30 days for transient occupancy. I was forced to move the boat to San Diego. I like San Diego a lot as a visitor destination, but I didn't care for it at all as a sailing venue. The winds are usually very light, the area is prone to thick fog and there really aren't any destinations accessible for just a weekend's cruise. I was too scared by the horror stories that floated around the docks about the paperwork nightmare of bringing a boat into Mexico to attempt that. Only Mission Bay remained as a close-by option, and once you've done Sea World, there isn't much more to see or do.

At about the same time, my lease-back to the Moorings was coming to an end. While I hadn't nearly as much vacation time with the new company, I tried to get down to the Caribbean as much as possible to maximize my final season aboard *Ad Ease*. Also about this time, a friend of mine told me that he'd had a good experience putting his boat in charter with an outfit based in Long Beach. I liked Long Beach as a sailing venue because it is the closest port to Catalina, where I loved to sail. Lacking any other viable options to obtain a suitable slip, and since I was traveling constantly with the

46

new company, it seemed like a good idea to put the boat in charter. By the time the Beneteau 51 finally sold, I was beginning to get a lot of resistance from my family to sailing. Both kids, now in school, had full agendas of their own and my wife and I both felt obligated to support them by staying at home on the weekends and being available for their activities. My marriage wasn't going well at this time and my wife and I ultimately agreed to divorce. I moved out of the house and found myself living in the same condominium project where I had temporarily lived several years before. I thought it would be a short-term arrangement, but my divorce was drawn out and complicated and I spent almost two years in that condominium.

Along the way, I was reintroduced to Sharon Nazari. I was in the resort development business and Sharon was the membership director of the American Resort Development Association. We had met earlier, but at the time we were both married. While we both unquestionably felt some instant attraction, we prudently backed away quickly. But once separated from our spouses, we could not possibly resist pursuing our attraction. It wasn't long before we started dating bi-coastally. I was doing a significant amount of work in both Florida and Cape Cod, Massachusetts, so it was convenient to stop in Washington on my way there or on the return trips. Sharon's daughter was in high school and there was no prospect for her to move, so we carried on this way for over a year. When I wasn't going east, Sharon would fly out for the weekend to California using my bonus miles.

When I was a young man, I remember reading somewhere, probably in *Playboy* magazine, that you should always perform a "linen test" before getting married. Given the sexual freedom that followed the Sixties and the more liberal attitude of the Nineties, this seemed like an unnecessary piece of advice. But because Sharon had never been sailing, I was equally interested in giving her a sea trial. So one cold, winter night after she had flown into LAX, I took her sailing to Avalon on Catalina Island. Sharon was a natural and when we got to the Island I almost had to rip the wheel out of her hand, because in spite of the 20-to-25-knot winds and the building six-foot seas, she was having a ball and didn't want the sail to end. This was all I needed to know. Then and there I resolved that when the timing was right, I would ask her to marry me.

After her daughter graduated from high school, Sharon moved to California. It didn't take her long to get a good taste of West Coast weather and the laid-back lifestyle that was in such contrast to her East Coast upbringing. She quickly grew especially fond of Catalina, sharing my love for the island, and we would sail there as often as possible. On one of our trips, near Christmas, I'd seen a flyer announcing that a movie we wanted to see was playing, so we went despite the gloomy weather. Only when we got there, it turned out that the local elementary school was having their Christmas show and the movie wasn't playing. Having made the hike in a driving rain, we decided to watch a little bit of it since we were already there. Trust me. You do not want to watch an elementary school Christmas show unless your own child is performing. After a time we started getting a good case of the giggles and had to make a hasty retreat before we disturbed the audience and embarrassed ourselves.

We were fortunate enough to attend the 1995 America's Cup regatta in San Diego during this time period. With the help of my friend Gary, who ran the charter company that had managed *Venus Butterfly*, I obtained a slip right in the America's Cup Harbor in San Diego. This was an amazing location and we could watch all the boats preparing to race in the morning and again when they came back at the conclusion of the day's racing. We were right next to the New Zealand compound, and of course, since they ultimately won the Cup that year, it was *the* place to be.

I'll never forget the trip down the coast to San Diego. We had to move the boat on a weekend. We left Long Beach quite late on a Friday night because before we could set sail, we had to position a car in San Diego. It was around 11:00 p.m. by the time we'd picked up my daughter, Whitney, and were able to set sail. Within an hour after leaving Long Beach Harbor the engine overheated. There was a very light breeze and the best we could do was to ghost along at two or three knots, aided by the knot or so of current that flows southeastward along this part of the California Coast. It was daylight when we got to Newport Harbor, so we decided to put in and see if we could find a mechanic. We stopped at the gas dock and they called a local mechanic who was good enough to make a special trip to help us out. He thought the problem was something clogging the raw water intake, so he cleaned everything out and sent us on our way.

We barely made it out of Newport Harbor when the engine overheated again. This time I made a thorough investigation and discovered a crack in the fresh water pump that was leaking air into the system and breaking the vacuum. With no spare pump on board there wasn't much that I could do to affect a repair. Since the weather was beautiful, we had lots of provisions and all weekend to cover the remaining 70 miles, we decided to push on. I made a couple of radio calls to other boats we knew were also sailing down to check on conditions ahead. The Coast Guard intercepted our traffic and suggested that we talk to Vessel Assist. Vessel Assist is to boaters what the Automobile Club is to drivers. We were members, so I thought that was good advice. They strongly tried to dissuade us from continuing on and offered to tow us back into Newport for repairs. Did we have enough food and water? Would our batteries hold out? After listening to all their admonitions, I told them I was confident that we could make the trip, but I did accept their offer to establish regular radio communications. For the rest of the trip I checked in with Vessel Assist once every four hours so they could stay aware of our position and situation.

This turned out to be a very slow trip. The wind barely blew at all the rest of that day, overnight and Sunday. We ghosted along at one or two knots, conserving all the electricity we could, so we would have house batteries for the overnight sail on Saturday, and as it turned out, most of Sunday night as well. I do remember this as an enjoyable sail, however. Sharon and I established a watch schedule to provide relief to each other and I managed to get a little sleep along the way.

Children are so cute when they are young. It was a little after midnight on Sunday when the wind finally started to blow. We were about 10 miles from the entrance to San Diego Harbor and Sharon and Whitney were both asleep. We suddenly went from no wind to about 20 knots. That was a big relief because by now I was exhausted, the batteries were getting low and I was anxious to make port. When the wind started to blow it also kicked up white-caps. There was an abundance of phosphorescent plankton in the water that weekend and all the whitecaps were glowing with that beautiful luminescent blue that plankton emanate when agitated. It was also particularly eerie because schools of fish looked like massive apparitions moving towards the boat. All the noise in the rigging as the winds picked up awoke my daughter. She came up on deck and asked me what was happening. I told her we had a strong wind and that we'd be reaching port within a couple of hours. She sat silently for awhile and then she said "Dad, can I ask you a question?" I said sure and in a voice that belied her attempt to project confidence, she said, "Dad, do you ever get scared?" With a straight face I told her that lots of things scared me, but sailing on the ocean wasn't one of them. That seemed to satisfy her and she went back to bed.

As we entered San Diego Harbor and started sailing towards Shelter Island and the America's Cup basin, the wind died again. I was getting a little worried about how I was going to make a land-ing. I had no clue exactly where the assigned slip was located and feared that the motor, which I'd need to maneuver, might overheat before we could safely dock. We ghosted into the basin and found the dock with our assigned slip. With no wind and a slight oppos-ing current, there was no way I was going to dock the boat, so I decided to chance running the engine just long enough to maneu-ver into the slip and get tied up. It would take the engine a few minutes to warm up before it would overheat, so I started it up. Fortunately I found the slip right away and made it in before the engine had time to overheat. We all slept well, but only for a few hours because we had to get to work and school, respectively, which required leaving early enough to get on the freeway before the rush hour traffic in San Diego and Orange counties. The races would start the following week and we had a vacation planned so that we could watch the entire series.

We had made arrangements for a number of guests to visit us for the races, making for a busy agenda. The two of us decided to watch the races by ourselves on the first day to get the lay of the land before we had to deal with all of the company. We motored out to the race course that first day and were somewhat surprised at the height of the seas. The swells were eight-to-10 feet. The race course consisted of a starting box around which all the spectator vessels took position and held station for the start. It was pretty unnerving, because in addition to the high seas, we often found ourselves parked next to huge spectator ships that towered above us and looked like they would crush us in the big seas if either of us made a mistake while trying to hold position. In addition, the competitors weren't bound to stay within the starting box, so occasionally they would sail on what we were sure would be a collision course, only to duck behind us to avoid a foul with their covering opponent. It was extremely exhilarating.

We soon realized that once the starting gun was sounded, there was no way we could keep up with these high-tech speed machines as they raced up the windward leg, so we decided to head back in and see what we could see on TV ashore. I got really lucky right at the outset and my Irish gift for the Blarney really paid off in spades. A local restaurant had been commandeered for the duration of the event to house the America's Cup Club, which was open only by invitation and limited to the syndicate members, race officials, local politicians and their staffs. When I heard about it, I thought about an old adage I had heard years before, "You don't get anything in life you don't ask for." So off we went to the America's Cup Club. By good fortune the owner of the restaurant happened to be at the door when we got there, and after engaging him in conversation for a few minutes, he must have decided we were okay people, because he issued us four passes right on the spot, two for us and two for the various guests that would soon be arriving. The really cool thing about this Club was that ESPN had set up a couple of dozen small television monitors around the room and we were getting the raw feed from the race course, commercial free. This was a great way to watch the races.

So one by one, our guests started to arrive. I knew my mother loved to sail, as did my daughter and her friend, but I guess the big seas and the proximity of so many large boats, all riding the swells in an undulating rhythm was too much for some of the others. Sea-

51

sickness is not a pretty sight. Meanwhile, we held station watching the "dance of the lead-bellied money gobblers," as world-class sailor, author and television commentator, Gary Jobson, described the jockeying for position at the starting line of a match race. These poor, seasick people all hung in there, probably out of deference to those of us who were healthy and wanted to watch the start. Sharon recalls trying to make lunch down below, while Pat, the wife of my attorney and friend, was sick as could be. Sharon felt so bad slapping sandwiches together while poor Pat was turning green and hanging on to the bucket.

Other than that, we really did have a sensational time. Ron happened to know a judge in San Diego who belonged to the San Diego Yacht Club and who helped us get a 10-day pass. The San Diego Yacht Club was the host venue for the event because they currently held the Cup. We were thrilled to visit the club and get some great photos with the Cup, particularly since that was the last time it was in the States.

During the week there were lots of other events, including a big boat series held between the huge mega-yachts that had been brought to San Diego for the Americas Cup series. We saw a number of people boarding the 100-foot-long yachts, so we thought they were open to the club members. We decided to have a look and thoughtfully kicked off our shoes at the stern, as we'd seen others do. As we started up the boat's huge broad staircase, we were immediately intercepted by three or four crew members. It turns out the boats were only open to the competitors in the event. We were politely, but summarily, invited off the yacht, with the explanation that the owner was back on board and the boat closed to company.

Later that night, while we were dining at the club, a debonair fellow wearing a smoking jacket and a white scarf made an appearance on the stern of the boat and literally took a few bows, mostly to the air and a few gawkers inside the club who happened to notice his arrival. Honestly, the scene was right out of an Errol Flynn movie and it was all we could do not to laugh out loud. Later we learned that the owner of the boat and personage who appeared on the fantail was none other than the Sultan of Brunei. The Sultan, who has held the position since 1967 is Hassanal Bolkiah Mu'iz-zaddin Waddaulah. Easy for me to say, right? The Sultan has a colorful history which has not been without controversy, including claims made in court proceedings by a former Miss USA and several girlfriends with whom she traveled that they were held as sex slaves for over a month by the Sultan and his associates. The suit was dismissed because the court lacked jurisdiction over the sovereign. The Sultan currently has two wives. He divorced one of his wives, a flight attendant, in 2003 and married a television personality in 2005. I'm sure he leads a very interesting life.

I have my daughter, Whitney, to thank for one of the most memorable experiences of our stay in San Diego. After watching one of the starts we were motoring back to the harbor when she spotted *Mighty Mary*, the nickname given to *America³*, a boat which had been sailed during the trials by an all female crew. She urged me to catch up with them. From the bow, my daughter yelled over and asked if she could come on their boat. Remarkably, they invited us to come to the compound for a tour. As soon as we got back to the harbor, we all piled in the car as fast as we could and made a bee-line for their compound where we were given a spectacular tour. Whitney and her friend were even allowed to haul a crew member aloft using one of the big "coffee grinder" winches aboard. I managed to capture a great picture of the two of them, which I later blew up to 11-by-14 inches and framed for her as a gift.

Riding back to our boat in the car we were chatting about what we had seen when Whitney, in one of those great kid moments, said "Dad, was that a big deal?" We all had a good laugh as we told her that it was indeed a big deal and that she really pulled off a good one talking her way onto that boat. It is surely one of the experiences that she will remember all of her life and as they say, "tell her grandchildren about," in years to come.

As the races proceeded it was clear that it was going to be a total rout. The New Zealand crew aboard NZL 32, dubbed *Black Magic,* clearly had the advantage in boat speed, tactics, and crew coordination, so it looked like it was going to be a clean sweep. As it got closer and closer to the end, more and more Kiwis started to flood into Shelter Island with each trans-oceanic flight. This was a lively, hard-drinking group and we got to talk and party with a number of them towards the end of the week. It was one of the most memorable party weeks I can recall in my entire life. The Kiwis were filled with excitement and pride and showed their enthusiasm in their good-natured, albeit rowdy, ways. As it turned out, Dennis Conner in *Stars and Stripes* was defeated 5 - 0.

Team New Zealand was headed by Peter Blake. We were moored adjacent to the Team New Zealand compound and we would see Peter Blake before each race as they headed out to the course and then at the end of the day when they triumphantly sailed back to their docks after each successive win. Tragically, we learned that Peter Blake had been killed by pirates in Brazil in December, 2001, during an environmental exploration trip in South America. It was a shocking and tragic end for this talented yachtsman who had twice won the America's Cup, as well as the Whitbread Round the World Race in 1989, and had been appointed a Knight Commander of the Order of the British Empire in 1995 for his services to yachting.

Since Sharon didn't know anybody in California when she first moved out, she wanted us to make some mutual friends. One summer shortly after she moved, we attended the Catalina Rendezvous, an annual gathering of owners of Catalina yachts that takes place at Two Harbors on Catalina Island. There we met a group of sailors who all owned Catalina 36s and belonged to what was then called Catalina Fleet #1. Catalina has a number of such associations for like-minded boat-owners. Fleet #1 was based primarily in Marina del Rey. Because I traveled so much, we didn't participate often in the meetings and other activities of this group. But we did enjoy the cruises that they sponsored, mostly to the various harbors and anchorages on Catalina Island. When the boat wasn't being chartered, we would try to participate. Catalina Fleet #1 was made up of an unusually eclectic membership and we forged many close friendships within that group.

In mid-1998 there was a real fly in the ointment. I was finishing a project I had been working on in Southern California and was offered an extremely lucrative job based in Phoenix to develop a number of vacation ownership resorts. It was too good to pass up.

Sharon didn't want to go to Phoenix and she suggested that I just commute back and forth to see her. Sharon is an extremely talented public relations and marketing professional and it wasn't too long after I moved to Arizona that a local company got wind that she might be coming to Arizona too. When they made her an offer she couldn't refuse, she decided the commuting idea wasn't such a great one after all and ultimately joined me in Arizona.

We fell into a pattern of catching an afternoon flight to Long Beach, hopping on the boat and sailing to Catalina. Neither of us really had our hearts in the Scottsdale community, where we were living after moving. We decided it might be a good idea to expand our social horizons in Southern California. Most of the Catalina Fleet #1 members belonged to different yacht clubs in the area, and at the urging of our closest friends within the group, we joined the Windjammers Yacht Club, which later merged and became the Santa Monica Windjammers Yacht Club. We also wanted to expand our cruising horizon and the added benefit of reciprocity with affiliated yacht clubs had enormous appeal to us as well.

Between these two groups there were lots of cruises, not only to Catalina, but to other ports up and down the Southern California coast. We had a really nice 13-foot Boston Whaler that we towed around behind our Catalina 36 as our dinghy and shore boat. Boston Whaler makes an extremely sturdy, small boat that is virtually unsinkable, because of its foam core. Ours was powered by a very zippy outboard motor and we had a great time with it. Not to mention, it got us out of some tight spots on more than one occasion.

The story of how we got our Boston Whaler is worth the telling, but Sharon told it best in an article she wrote for Catalina's owner magazine, *Mainsheet*:

"Whale Watching in the Nude"

By Sharon B. Drechsler

Such a provocative title might lead you to ask, "Why was she watching for whales, in the nude?" What circuitous trail of events had led me to this humble condition – shivering, naked, streaming wet, and yet, stubbornly vigilant?

This odyssey had its genesis two years ago when one of Dick's associates made a noble promise. The associate, Mike, is one of life's throw-backs to a better time, a better life, a time when men were men and a man's word was his bond. Anyway, I think that's how the saying goes.

Reader, you're not going to believe this, but I'm not lying. We were given – yes, that means free to us, no charge, just because Dick's that kind-of-a-guy person – a fabulous 13 foot, 4-stroke engine driven Boston Whaler (a Dauntless for those of you who are in the know). You see, during Mike's early days of starting a new venture, Dick had supplied him with some good advice that helped him get his business started. And one night, while in a jubilant mood, Mike swears on his honor that when he makes his first million, he will buy Dick his dream tender, a Boston Whaler! Two years go past and Dick and Mike's paths meander to different directions. Then, one recent night, Mike calls to ask where to deliver the boat! Honestly Reader, I'm not making this up, out of the blue, he called!

So it happens that Dick and I set out early to Shock boats to pick up our new tender. We spend the rest of the morning breaking in the new vessel as we drive it up the coast from Newport Beach to Long Beach to join *Venus Butterfly,* our Catalina 36. In honor of Mike's company, Turnkey Marketing, we call our beloved new addition the *Turnkey Tender.*

After reaching Long Beach in a little more than an hour and a half, (which gave our five-to-seven-knot-sailor-hearts a flutter), we hitch the *Turnkey Tender* to our sailboat's stern and we're off on a trip to Marina del Rey to participate in the Opening Day ceremonies at the Santa Monica Windjammers Yacht Club!

A brisk, March day with light wind, we raise the mainsail, but also supplement with the motor. Chugging out of the marina into the Long Beach outer harbor, we attempt to set the autopilot, only to discover that the wiring has frayed, causing it to malfunction. Dick digs through his

56

toolbox for his electrician's tools and no sooner sets about repairing it than 'Whoop!' Down flops the mainsail.

Somehow (now I'm not going to pin blame or name names here, although Dick asked me to use an alias for him), the snap shackle on the halyard has given way. Dear Reader, this happened to us once before when we had a faulty shackle – and I know what's in store. In desperation I begin suggesting various alternatives: "There's no wind anyway, so let's just motor." (I knew that wouldn't be acceptable). "Didn't you say there was a spare halyard?" (This is spoken in a tone similar to a sportsman asking a charging bear for another shot). "Do the words 'Vessel Assist' or 'Sea Tow' mean anything to you?"

No, nothing would do but we must engage the now-functioning autopilot, put the most light-weight and trim person (what a salesman) in the bosun's chair and crank her up to the edge of the stratosphere.

My pleas to at least return us to the calm of our nearby slip fall on deaf ears. "Don't worry," he proclaims confidently, "it's just as calm out here as it is in the marina." Spoken like a man with both feet on the deck, don't you think?

And so it is that I am strapped into a bosun's chair and unceremoniously cranked up the mast by the now-appearing "spare halyard." Reader, I must assure you that this is something you don't want to do in your lifetime, if at all possible. Disregarding my husband's well intentioned advice ("Don't look down"), I struggle to the top, grab the halyard, and freeze in time for about a century or two. Reader, it's an ominously quiet world up there. It's just you and a bird or two in the kind of silence that resembles a time warp. Slowly, you sway from side-to-side in a giant 90° arc. In a period in which Genghis Khan could have re-conquered the Eastern World, Dick eases me back to the deck. (Actually, Dick's engineer's mind took hold of him here, and he figures a speedy descent will put an end to his shoulder pain. I've still got friction burns on my thighs.)

57

Now here's the first of many valuable lessons we've learned from this trip: When you're retrieving a halyard from the top of the mast, be sure to stop at the spreaders on the way down. This handy little tip will help you avoid the necessity of having to be cranked half-way back up again to properly position the main halyard aft of the mast, where it belongs. So much for upward mobility!

This done and the autopilot behaving itself, we proceed up the coast for a time, the wind diminished to a zephyr. My husband harkens to the siren call of the Whaler. Here's where we learn another very valuable lesson: Once you begin a motor-sail, don't stop.

We slow down just enough for Dick to hop aboard the *Turnkey Tender*. The transfer complete, I crank up *Venus Butterfly's* motor to her normal 2400 rpm. No sooner is the Whaler cutting figure-eights through her wake, than the sailboat's motor starts spewing smoke like a truant puffing his first cigarette. *Venus Butterfly* was jealous. I couldn't blame her, I was feeling a little neglected, too.

Sure enough, our little pause to allow Dick to switch vessels was just long enough for the raw water intake to suck up a wad of seaweed, overheating the engine. It was evident that one of us had to dive under the boat (in minus-60-degree water) and clear up the problem. Unfortunately for me, I happen to be the only one with a wetsuit. With my heart in my throat, I dive a dozen times under the bobbing hulk of a hull, until at last I locate and clear the invasive blob. I emerge like a victorious plumber and tell Dick that he will just have to deal with any further problems. I'm heading for a hot shower.

We've now sailed and motored about half-way between Long Beach and Marina del Rey, to the Palos Verdes Peninsula and I've just peeled off my wetsuit and stepped into the warm, restorative shower when, sure enough, Dick spots a whale breaching. It must be a pretty awesome sight. It was certainly something I had whined about (or dare I say, wailed about?) wanting to see ever since moving to

58

Southern California. I bound onto the deck, dripping and shivering, only to watch a perfectly flat sea. It was about as much fun as watching water boil. No, it really wasn't that much fun, I've watched water boil.

And so it was that having swung from the mast and dodged the keel; in the end I was just another naked whale-watcher. Resembling a re-enactment of the Northridge earthquake, I shiver and wait in vain for this apparently truculent behemoth. I never did see the beast, but that's the story of the delivery of the *Turnkey Tender* and how I was reduced to whale watching in the nude!

If that trip wasn't calamitous enough, we would have one other problem. Shortly after arriving at the Santa Monica Windjammers Yacht Club, a couple of the guys came down to admire the Boston Whaler. Beaming with pride, I offered them a ride. We went all the way back out into the ocean so they could see how well it rode over the big swells, but when attempting to dock in a tight spot between the dock and the seawall, I clipped the prop on a rock and took a big chunk out of it. After only my first outing, I had to buy a new prop and send the other one in for repair, so I'd have a spare for many years to come.

We enjoyed our Boston Whaler to the fullest and it made a great fishing boat. I love to fish and fishing from the Boston Whaler was much easier than fishing from the sailboat. It was also great for towing kids on boogie boards and other sea toys. During one of the Catalina Fleet #1 cruises to Catalina Island, a giant water fight between boats had somehow ensued. We had brought a business associate of mine along, a daring sort of fellow who rode dirt bikes along mountain ridges and narrow cliff-side trails for 'relaxation' on the weekends. Once I armed him with a huge water canon and put him aside me in the Whaler, we set out to terrorize and assault the entire fleet. I think I was just lucky that the Harbor Patrol was nowhere in sight, for clearly our dangerous antics would have caught their watchful eye and led to a citation, or worse. This same friend temporarily dubbed her *Social Butterfly* during his visit, since we used her for visiting adjacent boats and attending functions ashore.

One summer we decided to take a trip up the coast to Morro Bay. Sharon had never rounded Point Conception and I was eager to broaden her sailing experience. As we were approaching Port Hueneme at the south end of the Santa Barbara Channel, a busy shipping lane, we were suddenly blanketed by zero-zero fog. We had a near catastrophic accident when a huge tanker loomed out from the fog on a collision course with us. I swerved and just avoided a collision. When I finished shaking, I resolved that it was time to put radar on the boat. Once safely in Santa Barbara, I looked up the local marine electronics shop and made arrangements to have a Furuno radar unit installed the next day.

Our rounding of Point Conception was uneventful and we put into Port San Luis for an enjoyable evening and visit at the local yacht club. The next day we left for Morro Bay and enjoyed a lovely two-day stay. The enemy of a cruising sailor is a schedule, but since we were on a limited vacation and had to get back, against the advice of the other local cruisers, we put out in the face of a forecast "California eddy." To tell you the truth, at the time I had no idea what that was. It didn't sound bad, and not having ever experienced this phenomenon in all my years of Southern California sailing, I thought, "How bad can it be?" and made the fateful decision to leave the safety of Morro Bay.

We were planning to retrace our route and put back into Port San Luis on the return voyage. However, only three hours out of Morro Bay, about the time we were passing the Diablo Canyon Nuclear Power Plant, the California eddy arrived, packing gale force winds that soon drove the seas to steep 11-foot monsters with breaking crests that threatened to drive the Boston Whaler up and into the cockpit, with potentially deadly consequences. While the autopilot was still holding the boat on course in the building following seas, I was able to put the Boston Whaler out about 200 feet on two lines that I rigged to form a yoke. As the following seas built to proportions that had the potential to pitchpole *Venus Butterfly*, towing the Whaler so far behind proved to have a beneficial consequence. The Whaler acted much like a drogue anchor -- a parachute-like apparatus that can be deployed for this very purpose. As we would start to hurtle at perilous speed down the face of the larger waves, the tow line would suddenly spring taught and slow *Venus Butterfly* just enough to let the offending seas roll harmlessly under her keel.

As the seas continued to build and the sky darkened, Sharon got very scared and began to cry, fearing for her life. While I knew the situation was under control, it did require my constant hand on the wheel because the seas were now way beyond the range of the autopilot's ability. I had to do something to try to reassure Sharon. Visibility was no more than 10 miles. Out of sight of land and with overcast skies, we had no point of reference but the compass heading, so I asked Sharon to go below to the laptop, which was running our GPS navigation program, and give me an idea of our position. Unfamiliar with the software, she accidentally activated the man overboard function, which caused the routing to freeze. Clearly, with darkness falling, in dangerous sea conditions and approaching a lee shore, I had to rectify this situation.

There was nothing to be done for it. I had to put Sharon at the helm. Crying the whole time, she assumed the helm and with me at her side, slowly adapted to the sea state and was managing to keep the boat in trim. After about a half-hour, satisfied that she would be okay, I darted down below. I looked for the biggest glass I could find, filled it halfway with ice and the rest of the way with Johnny Walker Black, Sharon's scotch of choice. Armed and ready, I clawed my way back to the cockpit and thrust the glass at her, with an order delivered in a tone not to be countered, "Drink this!" Well, a half-hour later you would think it was a scene from *Surfin' USA*. Sharon was having a ball and doing a yeoman's job of handling the boat. That freed me to restart the navigation. I realized almost immediately that any chance of reaching Port San Luis, which we had already passed, was out of the question. There was no choice but to push on past Point Conception to Cojo Anchorage, a small cove in the lee of Government Point.

I made a quick sandwich for dinner and as darkness settled in, I assumed the helm for the remaining five hours left to reach our destination. It was a grueling night with gale force winds and seas that made it exhausting and painful to hand-steer. But by about 11 p.m. we were rounding Point Conception and only two miles from

61

the relative calm of Cojo Anchorage. That's when it happened. We heard the loudest explosion I can ever recall. In the pitch black of the night I had no idea at first what had happened. I was reasonably sure we hadn't hit anything or the boat would have reacted. But all I noticed at this point was that we were slowing down slightly. A powerful flashlight aimed at the rig quickly revealed our fate. The mainsail had blown out, splitting cleanly along at least two seams. With the strong winds coming from directly astern, the shredded sail and control lines had quickly wrapped themselves almost inextricably in the shrouds, forestay and radar dome. I quickly started the motor, and after an excruciatingly long hour, we made our way into Cojo Anchorage and dropped anchor.

While we were completely sheltered from the seas, the winds in the anchorage were still blowing in the mid-20s with higher gusts, so I feared that leaving the sail in place could cause the anchor to drag with dangerous consequences. It was too dangerous to ascend the mast with the shreds flopping wildly, so I pulled the remains of the sail down as far as I could and climbed atop the boom where I cut the bolt rope as high as I could reach. Once I cleared what I could there was still a large piece of sail atop the rig that would flutter noisily all night long. Exhausted after nearly nine hours battling rough seas and confident the anchor was holding, I immediately fell into a deep sleep. Sharon, on the other hand, was convinced the anchor was going to drag and told me in the morning that she hadn't slept at all.

As rough and windy as it had been just hours before, when I awoke the next morning the skies were sunny and the Pacific Ocean resembled a lily pond. There was not a trace of the tempest we had fought the night before. Once we weighed anchor for the 40-mile motoring trip to Santa Barbara, Sharon went to bed. The dead calm seas made it possible for me to use the boat hook to clear out the rat's nest that was our mainsail. I also managed to get a call off to Gary at the charter company using the VHF radio-telephone operator service to see if he could offer any help. He put me in touch with a sailmaker in Santa Barbara. Long before we arrived, he had located a used sail in Santa Cruz, made arrangements to ship it overnight to Santa Barbara, and if everything went according to plan, install it the next morning so we could be on our way.

That evening, recovered from the ordeal and happy to celebrate being alive, Sharon and I enjoyed a wonderful dinner at one of the good restaurants that overlooks the Santa Barbara Harbor and its busy fishing fleet. The next morning, as planned, the sailmaker arrived with the sail and we were soon on our way, as if the whole incident had never happened.

It wouldn't be long before we were to put our radar to a real test. We were making a night sail from Marina del Rey to Long Beach, returning from a weekend function at the yacht club. The winds were blowing 15-to-20 knots and we had a fairly decent swell running, which coupled with the whitecaps and the fog, made the sailing fairly rough. Somewhere off the Palos Verdes Peninsula I noticed that the line holding the Boston Whaler had come loose and the Whaler was nowhere to be seen ("Now I'm not going to pin blame or name names here, although ~~Dick~~ Sharon asked me to use an alias for ~~him~~ her"). It took us a couple of hours, but with the aid of our newly-installed radar unit, we were able to find the Whaler. We were overjoyed that the radar had paid for itself during its very first sea trial. I would never sail without radar again.

The following few years were filled with the same routine. We'd fly out from Phoenix to the boat on weekends and vacations to participate in the various cruises and yacht club events. The highlight of our annual social calendar was the Catalina 36 Fleet #1 Christmas party. By this time, Fleet #1 had grown and included more than just Catalina 36s. Since so many of the members had moved up to bigger boats it was renamed Catalinas of Santa Monica Bay. At this Christmas party we played the gift exchange game where you could steal any gift twice. With this group you never knew what manner of off-beat gift you were likely to draw. One time before we realized we'd be breaking the rules, we bought something we knew we wanted, so we could steal back our own gift. Charlene, who ran the event with a steel hand, may have caught on to us, but was kind enough to turn a blind eye.

On one memorable occasion we took Sharon's daughter, Roxanne, and her friend Suzanne, sailing to Catalina. This was

Roxanne's first trip aboard *Venus Butterfly*. Roxanne was in college on the East Coast when Sharon originally moved to California and she'd missed the learning curve when it came to sailing. So Roxanne had no idea what to expect. Both girls took Dramamine to avoid getting sea sick and fell sound asleep below-decks. Sharon and I moored the boat to one of the mooring buoys and settled down in the cockpit with a cocktail to celebrate our arrival. Roxanne awoke first and poked her head out of the companionway. She was aghast as she looked around in horror and said "Suzi, you'd better get up here. There's no dock!" Sharon and I were beside ourselves with laughter and wondering what, exactly, Suzanne was going to do about it. On that trip Suzanne also lost a rented dive mask and snorkel and to this day the subject always comes up, much to her dismay, whenever we see Suzanne.

Earlier I wrote about learning to sail at the Catalina Island Boys Camp. One summer the charter outfit with which we were affiliated decided to throw a party for all the boat owners in the fleet at Howland's Landing. Mind you, I hadn't been back to this spot since going to camp there and learning how to sail as a kid. This was a tremendous opportunity and one I was bound and determined not to miss. I have some nearly-lifelong and very dear friends, Dan and Phyllis. Because they had spent many years working abroad, I'd not seen much of them. When they finally did return, I was living in Phoenix, so I would jump at any chance to get together. I am very close to the whole family, which has become my adopted family now that my mother and father are both gone. Because it was such a nostalgic outing, we decided to invite Dan and Phyllis to come along. It was early in the year, March if I recall, and because it was getting dark quite early, it was a cold night sail. Both Dan and Phyllis got pretty serious seasickness during the passage. About 11 miles from Howland's Landing it was obvious they'd had enough, so I suggested I put them in the Whaler and take them on ahead to shore, leaving Sharon to single-hand *Venus Butterfly*. I figured I'd drop them off and get back to the boat well before Sharon could make landfall. In spite of the choppy two-to-three foot seas, we managed to make good time. Both of them were instantly relieved to be on *terra firma*. The assembled group had a fire going, so they joined in and warmed up quickly. Worried about Sharon, I wanted to get back as fast as I could. As it was pitch black outside, I figured the running lights of a lone sailboat would be easy enough to spot once at sea. What I hadn't counted on was the fact that the backdrop of the bright city lights of Los Angeles made it all but impossible to pick out *Venus Butterfly*. Sharon and I had been in constant radio contact and I remembered that we had a 300,000 candle power handheld spotlight on board. I told her to dig it out and aim it right towards the island. That did the trick and I was able to home in on the light, making the round trip in less than two hours. The two of us enjoyed the rest of the sail on our own, arriving around 11:00 p.m.

Dan and Phyllis were more than ready to climb back aboard and get a good night's sleep by the time we arrived. Dan had learned that the next night there was to be a poetry competition, so he wrote a very clever poem about our adventures the previous night that earned him the hands-down vote for first place in the competition. Someone, maybe me, suggested that we tell some jokes. Well, joke-telling is actually my forte. I used to spend a lot of time dealing with bureaucrats during my land development days. I quickly learned that bureaucrats are pretty much a bored lot. I found that if I started every conversation with a new joke, maybe I wouldn't get what I wanted, but they would always take my phone call, which was half the battle. So I started off with one of my favorites, a short little tale about the Irishman whose wife falls out of the car on a drive to Killarney. When a cop pulls him over to advise him of his wife's plight he responds, "Oh, thanks be to God, I thought I'd gone deaf!" This joke-telling fest must have gone on for several hours and I never ran out of material.

In 2002 we would make another change. Now that we were living happily-married in Scottsdale and doing quite well professionally, we decided to take the boat out of charter. We wanted to leave a lot more of our personal belongings permanently aboard, since we usually had more stuff than we could carry on the plane anyway. My resort development business was doing well, so coupled with Sharon's income, we figured we could afford to give up the charter income. The boat was showing the wear and tear of the years in charter, so we decided that rather than buy a new boat and take on a boat payment, we would just redo *Venus Butterfly* from the bottom of the keel to the tip of the mast.

It turns out that the first thing that had to go was the name. Early during the winter of 2001 a yacht club friend, Norm, asked me if I knew what a "Venus Butterfly" was. He knew the derivation of our boat's name, so I thought that was an odd question. He didn't want to say more, but suggested a Google search was in order. When I learned what it was, my face visibly flushed and I was mortified. Suddenly I knew why, on several occasions, the San Pedro marine operator had refused to correctly identify our boat by name whenever I used the service and kept referring to the "vessel *Butterfly*." While Wikipedia correctly defines "Venus butterfly" as a fictional sexual technique which was first mentioned in an episode of the Eighties American television drama *L.A. Law*, for those of you as naive as we were, it is also the name of a sex toy designed specifically to please a woman. To add insult to injury, at the Fleet #1 Christmas party shortly after Norm's comment and the subsequent revelation, before the gift exchange, one of our other friends made a big deal of announcing to the hundred or so revelers that he had a present for us. You guessed it, a "Venus Butterfly." But the final straw was when our yacht club refused to list the correct name of our boat, inserting "Butterfly" instead of the full name.

So as part of the complete make-over that was taking place, we went through the entire process of a de-naming ceremony. (You know sailors are very superstitious about these things). We followed this with a christening party we held at Cat Harbor, during which we had none other than our whistle-blower friend, Norm, officiate. The boat was originally white with maroon trim and canvas, although the faded canvas was now more of a dirty brown color. That color was very stylish back in the early Eighties. That's a period I jokingly refer to as the "mauving of America," when designers thought everything should be in grayish violet or reddish purple tones. By this time Catalina had also come out with an entirely new color scheme and I thought I could increase the value of the boat by knocking-off the newer colors. We also redid all the canvas and the upholstery, varnished the entire interior, upgraded the electronics and added a new heating system. Being in the resort development business, I figured when I retired and went cruising, the boat would truly be my last resort. That seemed a fitting name, so she was re-christened *Last Resort*.

Not having our boat in charter made our trips a lot easier and all but eliminated the need to make car trips to haul stuff back and forth. One of our cruises that I remember well was our first trip to the Channel Islands. Catalina is one of the Channel Islands, but most people are referring to the northernmost group of islands located across the Santa Barbara Channel from the cities of Ventura, Oxnard and Santa Barbara, itself, when they refer to the Channel Islands. We were anchored in a beautiful anchorage that had turquoise water similar to the colors I had seen in the South Pacific, a most unusual sight in Southern California. While we were out exploring the shoreline of this anchorage, we were approached by a dolphin. Dolphins often play in the pressure wave created by the sailboat when we are cruising, so I thought this one might play too. I gunned the Whaler and sure enough, the dolphin quickly caught on and started playing in the bow wake, just mere feet from where we were sitting. This led to one of the most incredible encounters I've had with a wild animal in my life. For over a half-hour we continued this game, but throwing in increasingly complex tasks, including stopping suddenly and turning rapidly before accelerating away to effectively ditch the dolphin, which learned remarkably fast and soon began to unexpectedly break from bow-wave riding and speed away before submerging out of sight. Then, a few moments later, from beneath the Whaler the dolphin would splash to the surface and indicate it wanted to ride the bow wave some more. It was an experience I'll never forget.

On one cruise to Paradise Cove, a roadside anchorage located at the far west end of Malibu in the lee of Point Dume, we had the good fortune to catch a large California barracuda. This species of barracuda is notable because they do not sport the long, sharp teeth found in other barracuda around the world. This was a big fish and I hurriedly dumped it in the Boston Whaler so Norm could take my picture with it, since I didn't have a camera with me on this trip. We then went back and I quickly cleaned it so Sharon could prepare it for hors d'oeuvres to serve the whole group. When we got back to Norm's boat, a Catalina 42 where all the festivities usually took place because it was the largest boat in the fleet at the time, we were accused of substituting fish, because nobody could believe we could clean, prepare and cook a fish that fast.

For more than 10 years running, with only one exception that I can remember, it was our practice to spend Thanksgiving and partake in the holiday festivities at the Harbor Reef Restaurant at the Isthmus in Two Harbors. Two Harbors is a classic company-town and everyone there worked for Doug Bombard and lived in company-owned housing. There was always a good turnout of boaters and I would undoubtedly run into old friends and fellow-sailors for whom Thanksgiving dinner was also a tradition. The highlight of the evening was always the appearance of a troop of locals dressed in period Pilgrim and Native American costumes. One year, due to a weather forecast for inclement weather and strong winds, which can make the Isthmus a dangerous place to get caught, we all took the safe bet and went to Cat Harbor on the south side of the island. When the storm arrived, it fooled us all, because it came directly out of the south, the one direction that leaves Cat Harbor vulnerable to the seas. We spent one very long night and day while the storm made a direct hit. Norm's and another friend's boat, moored directly in front of us, literally played bumper boats all night long while the heavy winds stretched the mooring lines to the limit, allowing the boats to collide. The two of them spent much of the night positioning and re-positioning fenders in an attempt to avoid damage to either boat.

In 2003, in a truly fortuitous accidental discovery, I had my first experience with WiFi, or wireless fidelity, while visiting the Isthmus at Catalina. This is the technology that allows laptop and handheld computer owners to seamlessly connect wirelessly to the Internet at "hotspots." While hotspots are now located all over the country in restaurants, libraries, airports, bookstores and all genre of public locations, this was almost unheard of at the time. During 2003, my company, Vacation Development Concepts, had been awarded a contract by an affiliate of a large hospitality company to administer $27 million in matching grants for renovation projects spread across 70 of their vacation ownership resorts. WiFi was just beginning to gain popularity and I was getting hooked on it. It all started that year when we were moored at the Isthmus. I had recently bought a small handheld device on which I was running Maptech's navigation software and raster charts of Southern California. As I was playing with the device to program the route for our return trip on Sunday, a notification icon suddenly appeared on the screen telling me there was a WiFi network in range. Not having a clue what it was, I started following the yellow brick road, and before you know it, I was reading my email. Laughing out loud at this cool technology, I had to wake up Sharon to tell her about it, a moment that she still reminds me of to this day.

Suddenly addicted to the idea, I immediately purchased a new laptop that had a WiFi card and when I could, started to choose hotels based on whether or not they had WiFi. One thing I quickly discovered in my travels during this assignment was that the time-share industry was woefully behind in catching up to his technology. By this time about 50 percent of all hotels and all the Starbucks outlets had WiFi, but as far as I could determine, almost nobody in the timeshare industry as yet had WiFi.

Seeing an opportunity, I decided to explore this a little further. Because I had been in the timeshare resort industry basically since its inception, it occurred to me that I was uniquely positioned to introduce the entire industry to the WiFi technology and perhaps corner the market. I started researching with my computer and after several hours had located a few companies that I thought I might approach about some kind of a joint venture. This Google search led me to contact Jim, the owner and operator of Beach Wireless, located in Orange County, California.

I'll never forget my first conversation with Jim late in 2003. He told me that while there was nothing particularly mysterious about the technology, the hard part was to find locations in which to install a hotspot. I told him that I was either the best thing or the worst thing that ever happened to him, and after explaining what my company did and the contacts both my wife and I had in the resort industry, I boldly asserted that we could easily command the lion's share of the market if we moved quickly. After several more conversations we agreed to collaborate on a joint venture. I had my attorney draw up all the paperwork and started putting out some feelers. Because I was still president of The Plaza Resort Club Association in Reno, dating back to my days working for Bob Beaumont, this seemed like a good place to start. Jim and I actually met in person for the first time at the Phoenix Sky Harbor Airport, as I joined his connecting flight from Orange County on the way to Reno for our first site-survey. On that flight we signed the partnership papers and sealed our fate for the next few years.

Chapter 3
Life, Death and Something In Between

The year 2004 started out great. Business was booming. I was in the third and final year of a lucrative three-year contract to handle the refurbishment of 70 timeshare resorts owned and operated by one of the largest hotel chains in the country. My wireless Internet business, ResortWiFi, was going well too. If I had any complaint, it was that I didn't have much time for sailing. Sharon and I were both traveling a lot and only getting down to the boat every other month or so. But we were pleased to see our businesses doing well, so at the time I was content with the trade-off.

Several years earlier, I had been approached by a friend of mine, Alex, who was the president of a large resort management company. Alex had recommended my company for the job of administering $27 million in matching grants to perform refurbishments at some of the 100-resorts that his company managed. Like the job that brought me back to Southern California from Reno more than a decade earlier, this project came with a high degree of urgency. Alex knew my business was slow and that I had time to tackle an assignment of this magnitude.

Within a few days I had traveled to New York for an interview. I found the final interview with a former Senator, one of the Trustees appointed to administer the fund, to be an enjoyable, if not somewhat amusing, experience. I had a political background of sorts myself, having served in my early adulthood on the national campaign staff of the late Senator Robert F. Kennedy during his tragic run for the presidency in 1968. Shortly into the interview I interjected a question about the Senator's days in the Senate and from that moment on the topic of conversation switched and we had an enjoyable and engaging conversation about his experiences. I knew at that moment I had won him over. The rest was just a formality.

The early days of that project had been helter-skelter. It was exhausting, because I would usually visit three different locations at a time, which kept me airborne four or five days every week. As it happened gradually, I didn't realize the toll this routine was taking on my health. Being the guy with the check book, you can imagine that the managers at each of the 70 resorts included in the scope of the project went out of their way to wine and dine me. By the time the third year of this project rolled around, my weight reflected the abuse and I was tipping the scales at almost 250 pounds. My stomach seemed to be in a constant state of upheaval and the acid reflux disease that plagued me my entire life was in full bloom during this period.

And if I didn't have enough to do, the wireless Internet business I had started at the end of 2003 was doing very well and consuming what time I had left. I had a significant advantage when I started this company, because with my contacts in the timeshare industry, coupled with Sharon's intimate network established during her days as membership director of the American Resort Development Association, we calculated that we could corner the market before the competition knew the market existed. And of course, the 70 resorts benefiting from the largesse of the grants I was administering represented just the impetus I needed to establish the company, because they represented a full five percent of the total domestic market share in the United States and Caribbean. The success of ResortWiFi was destined to provide just the bridge I needed as the work for the trust began to wind down.

When we started ResortWiFi, most people had no idea what WiFi was. I remember somebody telling me that the first time he connected to the Internet wirelessly he giggled. I used that comment to my advantage in my sales presentation and I can't count how many times that was the exact reaction. It became a little easier to sell resorts on the need for a WiFi installation when I could point to the fact that one of the largest resort chains in the country was already installing WiFi networks.

During the summer of 2004, Sharon and I were counting our blessings and finally enjoying a much needed vacation aboard *Last Resort*. We were moored at one of our very favorite spots on

72

Catalina Island, Buttonshell Beach, but the peace and serenity this idyllic setting afforded would soon be shattered. A couple of days before we were scheduled to leave and return to Scottsdale, Sharon received a phone call from Bethesda Naval Hospital in Maryland, advising that her mother, Ethel, had taken ill and was in grave condition. Sharon was very close with Ethel, who was in fact her step-mother, and I could sense almost immediately that Sharon was not going to be able to endure the six-hour sail back to Long Beach and the overnight wait for a flight to Washington, D.C. Responding to the emergency, I radioed the Avalon Harbor Department and obtained a ferry schedule. Running the motor at full throttle, I estimated she could just catch the last ferry to the mainland, where it would be easy enough to transfer to the airport for a red-eye flight.

Her natural mother had died from breast cancer when Sharon was barely six months old. Sharon and I have always been kindred souls and I attribute part of this to the fact that we both lost a parent as infants. My natural father died from an accidental gunshot wound in traumatic fashion the winter of my second year. Sharing the pain of these untimely deaths suffered during our early childhoods had helped us forge the strong common bond that developed early on in our relationship. Sharon's dad, Scotty, a Colonel in the Air Force, had met Ethel in Montgomery, Alabama in the early Fifties, where she was also stationed as an officer in the Air Force Nursing Corps. He dated her for 20 twenty years before they ultimately married in 1967. The whole family adored Ethel and stayed connected with her even as the military stationed them at different bases and often, in different countries. Ethel was a constant source of strength and inspiration for Sharon and was really the only mother she had ever known, having been raised primarily by her grandmother and father. Sharon was extremely close to her and the fear and hurt I sensed when she first heard Ethel was taken ill tore at my heart strings.

After dropping Sharon at the ferry landing in Avalon, I secured a mooring buoy overnight so I wouldn't be single-handing the 22 miles back to Long Beach in the dark. The next morning I departed in the calm, flat seas for the return trip, an eternity during which I anguished for Sharon and worried about Ethel's well-being. Once the boat was secured in her slip, I caught the next flight back to Phoenix. Sharon, with whom I was back in touch by cell phone, had reported that while Ethel's condition was grave, it had stabilized. She said there was no reason for me to fly back there yet. Ethel's sister, Helen, was *en route* to Washington, D.C. as well, and once she arrived, if Ethel was showing improvement, Sharon intended to fly back to Phoenix, as she was due back to work in a couple of days.

Ethel stood all of about five feet tall, but anyone who underestimated her based on her tiny stature was always in for a rude awakening. Ethel was a remarkable woman, a firebrand who achieved remarkable success in life and served as a stellar role model for Sharon during her formative years. Ethel, like Sharon's dad, had achieved the rank of Colonel, and from her position as Chief Nurse of the Air Force, could have gone on to be one of the first female generals had she not retired from the military.

After Sharon returned to Phoenix, Ethel remained hospitalized and seemed to be steadily improving. Unfortunately, a couple of weeks later, she took a serious turn for the worse and word came that Sharon should return to Washington, D.C. posthaste. When she arrived she called to say that the prognosis was not good, so I dropped everything and caught the next plane out of Phoenix myself. Not long after my arrival, Ethel succumbed to a fatal heart attack, the culmination of snowballing complications and old age. Ethel was 86 at the time of her death.

Sharon was stoic during this time and took immediate command of the situation, organizing a memorial service at the local chapel in Leisure World, where Ethel and Scotty lived. Due to the number of deaths occurring in Iraq, the formal internment with full military honors at Arlington National Cemetery would not take place for another three weeks. I had been to Arlington National Cemetery on a previous occasion to pay my respects at the grave site of Senator Robert Kennedy, where an eternal flame burned as a constant reminder of what might have been, but I had never attended a military funeral before. To be buried with full military honors is one of the highest tributes a thankful nation can pay those to whom it owes a debt for their service and it was a majestic, albeit sorrowful event.

Unbeknownst to me, this was only the beginning of a three year journey that would test my very survival and cause Sharon to endure more personal pain in such a short time period than anyone should ever have to endure. While we were in Washington for the Arlington services, it became readily apparent that Ethel had done a good job of masking 91-year-old Scotty's failing mental faculties. Although we visited often, we were quite unaware of the depth of the problem. As Ethel's sister, who had been staying with Scotty in the interim between Ethel's death and the final services, had to return to her own home in Florida, Sharon stayed behind in Washington long enough to arrange for a day nurse to attend to Scotty once he was left on his own.

It was not long until it became clear that this arrangement would not be sufficient. Scotty had worsening dementia and had lost the capability to care for himself or to be left alone for any long periods of time, lest he fall down or otherwise hurt himself. After a lot of pleading and coaxing, Scotty reluctantly agreed to move into an assisted living facility in Fountain Hills, not far from our home in Scottsdale. With the aid of a geriatric consultant, we investigated several options and found this one to be the best available. It was a lovely place with lots of facilities including a bar and several dining rooms. I'll never forget Sharon's description of her father's first encounter there. He walked in, was shown around the place and taken to his new room, a clean, good-size one-bedroom apartment. After a few minutes he donned his hat and sternly instructed Sharon to take him to the airport so he could return to Washington, D.C., obstinately proclaiming that he'd seen enough. It took Sharon a long time to calm him down and get him adjusted to the idea of leaving his Silver Spring, Maryland home of 30 years. He stayed with us for a few days while we waited for the moving van, and once we moved him in he went peacefully, but not without a good measure of confusion and grumbling.

During the rest of the year we were occupied by frequent visits with Sharon's dad and our extensive travel schedules. Sharon was still working for the financial services company she had originally joined when she moved to Arizona a few years earlier, and although I had almost wrapped up the contract with the trust, I was now making frequent sales calls for ResortWiFi that had me traveling to and fro across the country. All of this took its toll on our sailing schedule and it seemed like an eternity between our increasingly less frequent trips to the boat.

But if 2004 had brought its share of pain and challenges, 2005 would only be worse. As I explained, in February, 2005, on what I thought would be a routine visit to the doctor to obtain treatment for a sinus infection, I was diagnosed with Stage III neck and throat cancer. My life would never be the same. I have already described the medical procedures and complications that followed earlier, so I won't dwell on those. That's not what is important now anyway. What is important is how I summoned the strength to fight the battle.

My doctors told me, both before and after my treatment, that neck and throat cancer is the most difficult and invasive cancer to treat. But even with all the warnings I would receive, I did not really know what was in store. Anyone who's dealt with the devastating news that they have been diagnosed with cancer can attest to the fact that you are immediately confronted with a multitude of options. One would think that the treatment options would be straightforward. To the contrary, patients are confronted with a myriad of options and asked to make immediate decisions, most of which the typical person lacks the skill or knowledge to make intelligently. Couple this with the fact that many early treatment decisions can have life-and-death consequences and must be made while many people are still in a state of shock, and often denial, and you'll begin to appreciate the conundrum. I have always been a hands-on, take-charge person, so confronted with this new challenge, I decided to confront it like every other challenge I'd faced in my life, by putting one foot in front of the other.

The first issue was the surgery. I was warned of all the possible complications to my throat, which included some difficulty eating, possible involvement of my larynx and ultimately my ability to speak, and in some cases, the ability to breathe normally. If a large number of lymph nodes, which serve multiple functions, including acting as filters or traps for foreign particles, serving as a drainage system within the body and as a reservoir for white blood cells, had to be removed, my immune system would be compromised. To what degree would be dependent on the number of lymph nodes they had to surgically remove. There was another complication that came as a surprise to me when I first heard it. It was likely, based on the initial test results, that the nerves that controlled my deltoid muscle would be contaminated by cancer and have to be severed. This would result in the inability to ever use my left arm normally again. I was told that it would be extremely weak and I wouldn't be able to raise it above my shoulder after the surgery.

I'd already done a fair amount of Internet research, so I thought I knew a lot. But the first thing I would learn is that cancer of the tonsils, where mine originated, is very rare and there is not a lot of literature available, at least to the layman, on the details of treatment. I knew that whatever it took, I wasn't ready to die. That resolve led me to the overriding premise of the decision-making process, telling the doctors to throw everything, including the kitchen sink, at me to cure this invasive plague. I remember the chemotherapist insuring me that he was going to do just that. But the decision to enhance the radiation treatment with chemotherapy was in itself controversial. My surgeon didn't think I needed chemotherapy and was pushing me to only have radiation treatment. The idea of using chemotherapy to enhance the radiation treatment in cases like mine is a fairly new concept and it seemed that there were as many available opinions as there were oncologists to consult. In an abundance of caution, I opted for both treatments.

The chemotherapy and radiation lasted about four months. I had radiation treatment every weekday for about a fifteen minute session. After about three weeks of treatment, my neck looked like I'd spent a week in the Malibu sun without sun screen. I was given every manner of balm and salve, but the skin would stay raw and excruciatingly painful for the remaining course of the treatment. Inside, my throat was similarly raw and I began to appreciate the feeding tube, even though I hated the inconvenience of being strapped up to it.

All of this was debilitating and I became increasingly weaker. I also suffered varying degrees of nausea. I became so weak that I couldn't climb the stairs at home. I also was required to take different drugs through the night. They were in liquid form or I would grind them with a mortar and pestle and pour them into the feeding tube. In order not to keep Sharon awake half the night and because I couldn't get upstairs, we decided early on to rent a hospital bed which we placed in the family room. I spent my days and nights in that room for the duration of the treatment, leaving only to visit the hospital and my doctors for treatments and examinations.

Luckily, we had finally seen our way at Christmas, 2004, to buy ourselves a flat screen high definition television set. I spent most of my time watching television. I remember watching a show called *Sunrise Earth* every morning as I patiently poured my first canned liquid meal of the day down the tube. The idea behind *Sunrise Earth* was to film an hour of sunrise at various spectacularly scenic locations around the world and enjoy the beauty and solitude in real time. A transformation of my values was beginning to slowly take shape. Up until the time I got sick, I had remained a political activist, although mostly from the sidelines and through my writing. Before this time, I had avidly kept up with public affairs and political news and had one of the three news channels, CNN, MSNBC or FOX tuned in almost 24/7. That began to change and I started to lose interest in all this news, over which I had no control and a rapidly waning interest. I recorded all the episodes of *Sunrise Earth* on the TiVo digital video recorder and preferred to replay the soothing natural sights and sounds during the day instead of listening to the constant barrage of negativity espoused by the cable news channels in their frenetic search for material to fill the news cycles.

I also continued to work as best as I could. My partner, while sympathetic, was shouldering most of the burden. Sales were slowing as it became harder and harder for me to work and for a period of about four weeks towards the end of the treatment, I lost my voice altogether.

78

I have always had a large circle of friends. I have an outgoing personality and make friends easily. As I also mentioned earlier, I have been blessed with the gift of gab, and if one believes the legend, it is obviously the result of kissing the Blarney Stone in Ireland at a tender age. I found that it was cathartic to write a short email each week to my close circle of family and friends, maybe 25 people, describing my treatment and the things that were transpiring at the time. I never saved those emails, which I regret.

It was during this time that an event occurred which not only bolstered my own hope for recovery, but planted the seed for some of the things I would do later. I received much positive feedback through my weekly emails and was inspired by the encouragement. One day Larry, a former business associate and close friend, emailed to say that his friend and neighbor had been diagnosed with cancer and had decided not to go through surgery or treatment, an effective death sentence. Concerned and alarmed for his friend, Larry asked if he could share some of my emails with this friend. By now I was finished with the treatment, but was still unable to eat and living the miserable existence I endured while tethered to the crippling feeding tube. I of course consented and Larry took many of my writings over to the fellow's house that night. After hearing my story, Larry happily reported that his friend had changed his mind and was going to consent to the surgery and treatment. Apparently the fellow made a comment to the effect that if I could go through all I'd endured, so could he. The fellow's surgery and treatment were a success. He had his bladder removed and has to live with a bag, but it could have been much worse. Mayo Clinic in Scottsdale now uses him as a resource to talk with and inspire men facing the same operation. He has recently celebrated his 80th birthday. This was the first time I would learn that I could provide inspiration to others.

I remember trying to go sailing a time or two while I still had the feeding tube in place. It took about 45 minutes to eat. I remember being underway in a good-sized sea swell and lying down in the cockpit trying to administer my food. I do not like to be out of control, especially as the captain of a ship in a busy seaway. Poor Sharon, I'm afraid I made her life miserable during this experience, barking orders out of frustration and complaining about everything she was doing at the helm. I seriously considered selling the boat at this time, but thankfully, at the urging of my friend Jim, an associate from Reno, opted to hang in there with it during this ordeal.

As more and more people learned of my plight, I was somewhat incredulous at the outpouring of sympathy and the amazement they expressed over my optimistic attitude in the face of the severity of my illness and my total inability to eat or drink. I guess I was learning to live with it, because it never seemed as bad to me as it did to those around me. Especially in Sharon's case, I thought it was far easier to be the one who was sick than the one burdened with the role of caregiver. And for Sharon, it wasn't just me that she had to contend with. By the end of 2005, her dad's dementia was getting worse, probably through the combination of old age and Parkinson's disease.

As helpless as I felt, it was made even worse by Sharon's professional circumstances. There had been management realignment in the company where she was employed. It wasn't working out well for Sharon and she was becoming unhappier as the days went by. I could tell all the stress of caring for both me and her dad, plus her difficulties in the office, were beginning to take a toll on her. So I watched as she endured all this and hoped somehow, some way, I could help ease her burdens before too long.

Meanwhile, my quest for a solution to the problem with my throat continued. During every spare moment I would research the problem on the Internet. I read of some doctors in Berlin who were experimenting with ways to treat conditions similar to mine. It turned out that more and more patients who elected to undergo both chemotherapy and radiation for similar cancer were presenting with varying degrees of stenosis (blockage) of the esophagus and the demand for some type of restorative procedure was growing. I also read about trials at the University of Pennsylvania that sounded promising. With each new discovery I would call my oncologist to consult with him on my findings. He is a dedicated practitioner, as well as a friend, who never gave up the search for a solution.

My oncologist called in early January, 2006, to tell me that he thought he had found a doctor at the M.D. Anderson Cancer Center in Houston who might hold the key to reversing the damage to my esophagus. The timing wasn't good however. Sharon's dad was deteriorating further. She was under increasing pressure to move him from the assisted living section of the campus where he lived to the skilled nursing area. This was going to be a painful decision and Sharon procrastinated as long as possible. Our consultant, Linda, who had grown very fond of Scotty during the past year, also had mixed emotions. She knew the move would signal the beginning of the end for Scotty and counseled that with some pressure on the nursing staff, she thought she could convince them to keep him where he was for a time.

I was finding it more and more difficult and awkward to work. Unable to swallow what little saliva I had, it would accumulate in my mouth, requiring me to frequently use a tissue to spit and swab out what I could. That was fine as long as I was working alone at home, but in business I was always being confronted with awkward situations at mealtime when unsuspecting clients and associates insisted I join them for a lunch or a dinner. Flying, it turned out, caused my throat to swell and close, so every time I went somewhere by air it was followed by a hospital stay requiring sedation to have my throat dilated. This grew old pretty fast.

Fortunately, my partner and I had agreed from the outset that when the time was ripe, we would try to sell the company. WiFi was getting very popular and we were just big enough that we were becoming not only noticed, but also somewhat of a thorn in the side of a few of our largest competitors, several of whom had now discovered the timeshare industry and were assaulting our market with a vengeance. I think the final straw was when one of our competitors began offering free installations. We simply did not have, nor did we have the wherewithal to raise, the amount of capital it would take to finance the multiple installations we were still doing each month if we had to perform them at our expense. We had also tried, with very little success, to branch out into other markets and were again hampered by our inability to raise capital. It was time to sell.

During the end of 2005, there was a flurry of activity as we weighed one proposal against another. Ultimately, we decided to close a deal with Wayport, our largest competitor. As part of the transaction, I signed a short-term consulting contract. I was effectively being forced into retirement. I was terrified by the prospect and as much as I wanted to retire, I had no idea what I would do with myself. I still had some modest consulting income from the Beaumont companies, but that was all. I wasn't even old enough yet to qualify for Social Security benefits, but Sharon was making good money and we thought we could make it. We concluded the agreement in principal and went through an exhaustive 60-day due diligence period, with the sale scheduled to close in January, 2006.

Juxtaposed against all the merger activity was the possibility that the doctor in Houston, who my oncologist had spoken to, could do something to at least partially rehabilitate my throat. In mid-January 2006, just before the Wayport transaction was scheduled to close, I traveled to Texas where the ground-breaking procedure to open my throat would be performed. The lead doctor in my case had performed five successful operations on patients with similar esophageal stenosis. I would be number six. As I described earlier, there wasn't going to be much of a recovery period because the surgical procedure, although experimental, would only have been problematic had my esophagus been punctured or torn in the process of opening and dilating it. Since the surgeons had taken great pains to ensure that this didn't happen, I was fully healed and consistently drinking liquids within a few days of returning from Texas.

The surgeons in Texas and my local gastroenterologist worked out a year-long regimen that involved repeated throat dilations every four-to-six weeks. The goal was to try to restore my esophagus enough that I could at least swallow soft foods. It was a long-term prospect and I was just happy to be living a more normal life. I was soon liberated from the abominable feeding tube.

Meanwhile, Sharon's life was becoming increasingly difficult. Things in her company were reaching critical mass. She was becoming unhappier by the day with the new management structure at work and it was taking a toll on her. She wasn't sleeping at night and her usual good humor was giving way to a short temper.

She was also worrying more and more about her dad and it was clear that she would have to consent to the pressure the assisted living facility was putting on her to move him to skilled nursing. During one business trip early in 2006, Sharon received a call reporting that her dad had experienced a number of small seizures and that his ability to care for himself, even to walk or get in a wheelchair, was so impaired that there was no choice but to move him. Sharon immediately dispatched Linda, our consultant, to assess the situation, and when she reported that it was time to make the move, we sadly agreed. I went to the facility to clean out Scotty's apartment and oversee the move. Hoping against hope and not wanting to upset Scotty, we put most of his things in storage. During the preceding year he had finally agreed to sell his house, so Sharon had spent a couple of weeks in Washington, D.C. at the time selling what she could, throwing out a ton of stuff, and shipping good things and keepsakes to Phoenix, where we had already secured a storage facility. It was therefore an easy matter to move his present furnishings to storage.

June and July created a firestorm. Late in May, the owner of Sharon's company and she were discussing the fact that Sharon was obviously unhappy. They mutually came up with the idea that Sharon might be happier if she quit her job and started her own public relations and marketing company. Her last day in the office was just a few days after that discussion, on May 31, 2006.

Shortly before her father's birthday on June 6, he took a sudden turn for the worse and died. Thankfully he lived long enough for the entire family to gather at his bedside and be with him when the time came. On the advice of a friend of ours, we had brought in a caregiver from a local hospice. Her presence and candid description of the events occurring during Scotty's final hours were very comforting. He died quietly in his sleep. During his lifetime he had been loved and revered by all those he touched, and the staff where he spent his final months was no different. As hardened as I thought they must be to death, with which they were constantly confronted, I was impressed at the outpouring of their emotions.

83

Scotty had also distinguished himself in the military, and like Ethel, had obtained the rank of Colonel by the time he retired. Scotty met Sharon's birth mother, Barbara, a school teacher in Arlington Virginia, while he was stationed at the Pentagon after the war. Sharon was born in a military hospital in Washington, D.C. and lived in a number of different places, which is probably why she retains her wanderlust.

Over the fourth of July weekend, in an attempt to get some respite from the recent events, we sailed over to Catalina and again moored at our favorite spot, Buttonshell Beach. I'd first discovered this tiny little cove when my daughter, Whitney, and I attended an Indian Princess weekend there at the YMCA-operated Camp Fox. Whitney had been delighted at the prospect of bringing a couple of her friends over on the Catalina 36. There was a very funny moment when Whitney and I were rowing along in my dinghy with a group using the camp's dinghies. One of the girls asked me how we'd gotten the dinghy to the island. With a straight face, I told her we'd rowed from Long Beach, 26 miles distant. That kid's mouth dropped until I finally told her the truth that we'd towed it behind our 36-foot sailboat.

While there, we started philosophically discussing our future. Sharon had launched her own business and right out of the starting gate had enough work to keep her busy and making almost the same money her former job had paid. I had concluded the sale of ResortWiFi and was retired. Because I had frugally saved a fair sum of money during my career, the significant windfall resulting from the sale of ResortWiFi, coupled with a modest inheritance from Sharon's dad, meant we had a new freedom we hadn't experienced before. I had always dreamed of buying a large sailboat and going cruising. The more we talked about it, the more it seemed possible.

There were lots of questions and issues. To begin with, what would we do with our house and our worldly belongings? We would need state-of-the-art communications because Sharon wasn't about to abandon the prospect of nurturing and growing her newly-launched business. She needed to be able to seamlessly communicate with her clients as if she was in her office. It all seemed daunting, but by the time the weekend was over a plan had

84

emerged. We had set a budget for a boat, new or used, and the search began. I approached this plan like I approach everything, by once again putting one foot in front of the other. I'm a big believer in the old saying that "a journey of a thousand miles begins with a single step."

My friend Gary, who ran the charter outfit we had previously worked with, had now become a yacht broker, so in addition to his duties running a large fleet of charter yachts, he found time to buy and sell boats for other people. He was doing okay at this branch of his business and had made good contacts with many of the local yacht brokerages. One of them was the Catalina Yacht Anchorage in Marina del Rey, an in-house brokerage owned by Catalina Yachts. When I called Gary and explained what I wanted to do, he was all over it like white on snow. It didn't take half a day before he called me back to enthusiastically tell me that the Catalina Yacht Anchorage had a Catalina 470 in their inventory that they were getting anxious to sell and were willing to deal.

Buying a new boat from a dealer had the instant advantage of solving two serious problems we would have had buying a used boat. First, they were in a position to take our existing Catalina 36 in trade, and second, because of a severe shortage of slips, especially a live-aboard slip which we needed if our plan was to come to fruition, I could make the deal contingent on the broker finding us a suitable slip in Marina del Rey. The boat in question was a Catalina 470. I was unfamiliar with this particular model, but because of my long-term relationship with Catalina yachts, I decided to pursue this option. I did a quick search of the Catalina Yachts website and what I saw when I clicked on the page with photos of the Catalina 470 dazzled my eyes. I quickly showed Sharon the pictures, and in truth, the decision was probably made at that moment.

During the negotiations, the dealer originally offered almost $10,000.00 less for the trade-in of our Catalina 36 than the blue book value of comparable Catalina 36s I'd seen advertised for sale. This was attributed to the age of the boat, the fact it had been in charter and the number of hours on the engine. Of course, this offer was made sight unseen, without the benefit of a survey or an inspection of the boat. We had a couple of ace cards. Even though the engine had 3600 hours, it had been under the care and maintenance of only one, exceptional mechanic in Long Beach. Except for the first year in San Francisco, the mechanic had a complete record of all the work that had been performed on the engine. On top of that, over the preceding few years we had poured almost $20,000.00 into the boat to upgrade, rename and repaint her. As a result and almost as a lark, in March, only a few months earlier, we had entered her in the Santa Monica Windjammer's Yacht Club Bristol Boat Competition. This was an annual competition usually won by whoever could bribe the judges with the best booze and hors d'oeuvres following the Opening Day in Marina del Rey ceremonies held at the club to commemorate the beginning of the sailing season. Armed with that advice, Sharon had prepared some lovely treats, but mostly we relied on the big bottle of Johnny Walker Black Scotch that we had purchased for the occasion.

We really didn't think we had a chance of winning, but it was a lot of fun. Ours was the first boat they inspected and by the time they were finished and ready to move on to the next boat, at least one of them was already "three sheets to the wind." Non-sailors usually think that a sheet is a sail, but in fact, a sheet is a rope, or line, that controls the sails. If three sheets on one of the square riggers of ancient days were loose and blowing about in the wind, then the sails would flap and the boat would lurch about like a drunken sailor, hence the derivation of the term. Much to our surprise, later that night at the club when the awards were handed out, we won Best in Competition. Little did we know that the award certificate we won and proudly framed and mounted prominently aboard *Last Resort* would be worth $10,000.00! But, sure enough, this became a pivotal selling point.

I know boats and I've owned more than half a dozen of them, all sizes and types, but I have to admit when I boarded the C470 for the first time I went into 'overwhelm.' Suddenly, I was confronted with systems and options with which I had little familiarity, things like bow-thrusters, long-range communications, an in-mast furling mainsail, a watermaker, hydroponic diesel heat and the like. Sharon and I both agreed that a new boat would be the best of all

86

the possible options and we signed away a good part of our fortune that day as we planned to pay in cash. None of this would have been possible were it not for the sale of my company, which provided sufficient funds to buy the boat and leave something left over to pad our nest egg.

The next phase of the process would be commissioning the boat. We didn't know what an undertaking lay ahead of us and at that time we were filled with excitement and joy at the prospect of actually owning a boat capable of transporting us anywhere in the world. Suddenly, our sailing horizon, which with few exceptions before this had been limited to the 200 miles of coastline between Point Conception to the north and the Mexican border to the south, expanded to include virtually the entire planet. It wouldn't be long before we were buying cruising guides covering everything from the west coast of Mexico to Skagway, the northern terminus of the Inside Passage in Alaska.

In spite of my near brush with death and the resulting handicaps, which included my throat and inability to eat any food except liquids, the partial disability of my left arm and shoulder, not to mention a compromised immune system, we were about to escalate our lives to a whole new dimension of exploration, excitement, adventure and risk. And while Sharon would continue to work, it would soon be from a makeshift office aboard a brand new 47 foot sailing yacht.

We have to confess that when it came time to pick a name for the new boat, we were stumped. We've stumbled across some names since then we might have chosen, but at the time we were still in love with the name "Last Resort" and we decided to keep the name for the new boat. We didn't like the idea of "Last Resort Two" or "Last Resort II," since either version seemed like a contradiction in terms. So we wrote into the contract that the dealer would have to completely remove the old name from the Catalina 36 before reselling it. Because sailors are very superstitious about these things, I actually performed a short de-naming ceremony in the presence of the delivery captain who would sail her away with his daughter, who was helping him on the day Bob, our dealer, had the Catalina 36 moved from Marina del Rey to his Channel Islands

Harbor office. The boat must not have liked that idea at all, because after years of almost trouble-free service, the motor died about six miles from the destination and the delivery captain had to arrange for a tow to get the boat into port. They say it was the result of sludge from the bottom of the fuel tank getting agitated in the heavy seas that day and clogging the fuel filter, but I attribute it to more than that. In any event, my pride and joy for the past 17 years was gone and we were officially without a boat since it would be several months at least before the new *Last Resort* was commissioned and ready for delivery.

Chapter 4
Delivery Day, Olé

Commissioning a nearly-50 foot boat with the capability to travel across the oceans and seas of the world is every bit as daunting a task as it sounds. Once the decision was made to buy the boat, a contract signed and the deposit paid, we were entering the next phase. The learning curve during the next six months was steeper than that of many of the classes I took back in college.

There were really four categories of equipment to consider. The first was the basic boat, the hull, standard rigging and basic electronics that come with a stock boat. Next there was the equipment we originally elected to install, naively thinking we would be finished. The next category included items that didn't work and which we had to upgrade or replace, and finally, there were a number of things we discovered we needed during our shakedown cruising over seven months in Mexico.

The basic boat was actually quite well equipped for anyone planning day or weekend sails in any of the popular cruising grounds around the country. It has such a beautiful interior, in fact, that it was profiled in an issue of *Architectural Digest*. Beyond the basic equipment, I had to start adding safety, navigational and other systems to suit our plans. There were three criteria that had to be met. First and foremost, the boat needed to be equipped for long-range cruising. Second, since my wife needed to continue to work and wanted to grow her business, we needed complete, state-of-the-art communications and a computer network with printing, scanning and Internet capability. And finally, since this new boat would be home for many years to come, it needed the same comforts as our home, which included a washer-dryer, central heating and air conditioning, as well as a home theater system.

I'm a big believer in spare parts. While I'm handy, I'm no mechanic, although I can fix a number of simple engine problems, especially those that relate to fuel or cooling. My theory is that it's always possible to find someone who can work on an engine, but finding the parts in foreign ports is usually impossible and shipping parts into a foreign country is always a headache of varying degrees, ranging from mild to migraine, depending on where you are. So I asked the local Yanmar dealer to make up a spare parts kit. I now carry a complement of spare parts that one mechanic commented "would be the envy of most Yanmar dealers." I have a similar kit for the Fischer-Panda generator, as well as essential parts for many of the other systems aboard *Last Resort*.

When you start installing electronic, navigation and communication systems, that's where the fun and expense begin. Let me start with the navigation systems. For as long as they have been making navigation software for laptops and computers, I have relied on Maptech's products, and it was to be no different when we were commissioning *Last Resort*. I originally chose Maptech and still rely on them because they were the first to utilize raster images of the actual National Oceanic and Atmospheric Administration charts, which are now available free online. I rely on their Chart Navigator Pro software for all planning functions, in addition to maintaining a database of over 2000 waypoints, into which I have transcribed descriptions from all the available sources, including cruising guides, the Coast Pilot and even a Google search now and then. The original choice for a ship's computer was a Hewlett-Packard Slimline which fit perfectly in the compartment at the navigation station and operated on Vista. I also use an electronic log book, Ship's Log Deluxe, which allows me to keep information on thousands of waypoints, a complete record of all passages, an inventory, as well as a fuel log and maintenance record, including all costs. The inventory function alone is worth the small cost of the software. With almost 2000 spare parts aboard, it would be virtually impossible to find a small part, especially under the stress of an emergency, without this electronic aid. The computer is connected to a global positioning system ("GPS") which is integrated with our Maptech chartplotting software.

I also installed an Automatic Identification System ("AIS") receiver. All ships over 300 tons are now required by the Safety of Life at Sea ("SOLAS") treaties to carry a Class A transponder. Much like an airplane transponder, these devices display a ship's course, speed, heading, name, call sign, size, destination, and most importantly the Closest Point of Approach ("CPA") and the Time to Closest Point of Approach ("TCPA"). I have found this to be an invaluable piece of equipment and I will frequently radio large ships and ferries, well in advance, to make passing arrangements or to inquire about their intentions and make them aware of our presence. While Class A transponders range in price from $3000.00 to $5000.00, plus installation, I was able to buy a SITEX "Black Box" receive-only unit for under $200.00 and by adding a Smart Radio electronic antenna splitter, I avoided the cost and inconvenience of mounting a secondary VHF antenna. The Federal Communications Commission has recently approved the Class B transponder for recreational boats to broadcast their own positions and the initial pricing is around $1000.00.

The primary navigation system aboard ship is a Raymarine E120 chartplotter, to which we added a Sirius radio weather broadcast module. I would have preferred to have the AIS receiver sold by Raymarine, so the AIS display would be available in the cockpit, as well as from the navigation station. At $1000.00, though, I thought the cost was unwarranted, especially with Class B due out within a year or two. We also added the LifeTag system to our array of safety equipment. This radio-based system consists of a wristband radio transmitter and a receiver mounted at the navigation station. If a crew member wearing this device should go overboard, the device sets off an alarm that immediately marks the person's position on the chartplotter and establishes a course heading and distance to aid navigation back to the person.

Since our crew scheduling is such that Sharon, who I call the Executive Officer or "XO" aboard *Last Resort*, generally sleeps through the night while I take the watches during hours of darkness, this seemed like the most important piece of safety equipment we could have aboard ship. But if I've learned anything in my many years of sailing, and reinforced by our voyage to the frigid, freezing waters of Alaska, it is this — never, never, never ever fall overboard. When cruising offshore at night aboard *Last Resort*, nobody leaves the safety of the cabin below decks without a safety harness, whistle, strobe light, Life Tag bracelet and life jacket.

I should interject that we had much discussion before settling on the title "executive officer," because we felt "first mate" didn't give Sharon enough credit for the duties she fulfills aboard ship and the other term commonly used, "admiral," seemed patronizing and unrealistic. But what really sold us on this title for Sharon was the plaque we read on the wall of the executive officer's quarters on the USS *Midway* when we toured her in San Diego:

The Executive Officer

> The roles of the Executive Officer, or "XO," are varied and complex. In addition to being second in command, the XO is responsible for the day-to-day activities throughout the ship as well as the cleanliness aboard. The XO oversees the administration of the command and is the primary screener of disciplinary cases prior to their being heard by the Captain. The XO is the senior officer of the wardroom mess. For this reason, his living quarters are some of the best on the *Midway*.

While the XO aboard *Last Resort* is responsible for the same duties as outlined above, she counts on me for all but the basics when it comes to operating our sophisticated navigation systems. We have our Raymarine chartplotter set up so that it can be viewed on the 45-inch plasma-screen TV mounted on the forward bulkhead of the main salon. In combination with a secondary keyboard and a portable remote autopilot control, it is possible to pilot and navigate the ship from the navigation station. The radar display on the plasma TV is far superior to the Raymarine 12-inch display in the cockpit and I've found on long overnight passages, especially in inclement weather, heavy seas or fog, it is much more comfortable to maintain watch at the navigation station with frequent trips up the companionway every few minutes to watch for any ships that might escape radar or AIS monitoring. Keeping a visual watch is critical at all times, but it is especially important in Mexico where small fishing boats, locally known as *pangas*, often venture far offshore at night and might easily contain a sleeping crew of weary fishermen. And any of you who have used radar know all too well that in rough seas, even another sailboat can be lost in the background clutter of large swells or rain.

One of the primary concerns Sharon expressed, and a crucial factor in her decision to venture offshore and into international waters, was her ability to effectively communicate so she could continue to conduct her public relations business. Therefore, we installed and maintain a state-of-the-art, yet affordable, communications system aboard ship. Communications are divided into voice and data, although they overlap when using voice over Internet provider ("VoIP") technology such as Vonage or Skype, the sailor's choice. For voice communications we use Verizon cell phones with global plans and a satellite phone. We also experimented with using VoIP, which worked moderately well with the WiFi network at the Coral Hotel in Ensenada, Mexico, which would be *Last Resort's* first port, although the Internet service tended to degrade late in the day when returning guests overburdened the available bandwidth. We also have an ICOM M602 VHF radio for local communications and an ICOM M802 single sideband high frequency radio for marine and ham radio communications. We both obtained our general class ham radio licenses before leaving for Alaska.

For data, our primary source is high speed WiFi service, when available. We have found in British Columbia and to some extent, in Alaska, that reliable WiFi service is usually available in the larger marinas for about $10.00 a day, or $30.00 a month for long-term service. We mounted an 18 dBi WiFi antenna which has a range of well over a mile. We use an Engenius USB adapter and WiFi card connected to the ship's computer by "active" USB cables. A standard USB cable only has an effective range of approximately five meters, so to boost the signal over the required distance we employed several "active" USB cables.

When WiFi isn't available, we have Verizon USB Aircards. These work well almost anywhere in the United States and Canada where there is cell service and are fast enough to support large attachments. On our voyage up the Pacific Coast, we were somewhat amazed to find that there were very few areas where we didn't have cell service. As we maintained a link with Norm, our friend in Southern California who was kind enough to monitor our progress on all of our passages, this was a great convenience.

Additional data options include a Pactor III USB modem which supports both Sailmail (a paid email service) and Winlink (a free service utilizing the amateur radio bands, but not available for any business use). The Iridium satellite phone also has a modem which supports data. We use the Ocens IP service to access the Internet via the satellite phone, although none of these last options have enough bandwidth to support sending or receiving other than the smallest attachments, mostly GRIB files and weather reports. (Gridded Binary data files are output files generated by computer forecasting models.) We recently added Inmarsat's Broadband Global Access Network ("BGAN") capability, now that satellites launched in late-2008 provide worldwide coverage. The addition of the Sirius weather module for the Raymarine integrated system was also a huge plus. That system displays weather radar, cold and warm fronts, storms, precipitation intensity, winds and seas, as well as marine weather forecasts and tropical weather alerts. It displays all this data, including automated buoy and weather station reports, directly on the Raymarine chartplotter.

In order to accommodate all the antennas we would require for our communications systems, we installed a Garhauer-manufactured stainless steel pole on the stern swim platform on which we have mounted seven antennas. I like to ask other sailors if they can guess what all those antennas are for and I often see people wandering down the docks trying to figure it out as well. The antenna array supports the Raymarine 125 GPS receiver, the Iridium satellite phone antenna, the WiFi antenna, a weatherfax-type antenna that supports digital selective calling ("DSC") service transmissions on the single sideband radio, a 2-meter external antenna for my handheld ham radio, the Sirius weather module antenna and a SeaTel gyro-stabilized satellite television dome. We finally have *our own* BRT ("big round thing") like I first saw in the Caribbean so many years ago!

We were installing a lot of systems with which I was unfamiliar. Early on, the rigger had to take a few days off to attend to another boat and I told the broker I wanted to spend two days aboard, alone with the owner's manuals, a stack of binders and booklets that consumed two garbage-sized bags and stood more than two feet high when stacked on the table. I came aboard and literally read each manual cover to cover and looked at all the plumbing, wiring and controls until I was comfortable with the boat and equipment. This helped to a large degree, although hands-on usage and the experience that resulted after tackling some of the system failures that would come later are what I primarily attribute to my ability to quickly identify, and in most cases, repair issues that arise.

Someone once jokingly wrote that life aboard a cruising sailboat consists of performing maintenance in strange, isolated foreign ports. We would find out just how true that was soon after leaving the dock for the first time.

It seemed like forever, but eventually November 14, 2006 rolled around. We were filled with excitement. We had already moved all of our belongings from the Catalina 36 to the new boat, so we only had the personal belongings we brought with us, plus the provisions we would buy before departure, to load when we arrived. At one point, I had a pre-commissioning checklist of over 50 items, but as the actual day drew closer, things were happening at an accelerated pace and the list was down to a handful of items.

Being out-of-state residents living in Arizona, we qualified under then-current California law for a sales tax exemption if the actual yacht delivery occurred outside of the state and the boat was kept outside of California for six of the first 12 months following the purchase. In an abundance of caution, we hired a law firm in San Diego that was familiar with these requirements to assure that all the t's were crossed and the i's dotted, as there was a significant amount of money involved.

As the dealer frantically attended to the remaining items requiring completion before we would take delivery, we spent the preceding weekend pre-positioning two cars in Ensenada, Mexico, where we were going to be moving the boat. Our close friends, Norm and Charlene, were going to join us for the cruise to Mexico, so not only did we need to move our car to Ensenada, but they needed a car in which to return, so in a three-car caravan we headed across the border.

The Coral Hotel Marina is well-known as the home of the "90-Day Yacht Club," so dubbed by Captain Lonnie Ryan who wrote a book about the area and what was to be expected when staying in Ensenada. This marina was a favorite choice of those choosing to comply with the old 90-day rule imposed by California at a time before the desperate need for additional revenues forced the state to rethink the rule and extend the requirement for California residents to keep a boat out of state for a full year. The manager of the Coral Hotel Marina is an affable chap named Fito. Educated in the United States, Fito speaks flawless English and runs the marina operation at the Coral Hotel with an efficiency not usually experienced in Mexico. After we selected a slip and paid the security deposit and first month's rent, there wasn't much left to do so we decided to head back to Marina del Rey.

Finally the big day arrived. The plan was that Bob, the manager of the Catalina dealership, would take the boat out to a predetermined location and Sharon and I, together with our salesman, would be ferried to the coordinates aboard a Vessel Assist boat. Our attorney had advised us that in order to comply with the letter of the law, we couldn't be on the boat until it was in international waters and using a private company provided the extra advantage of third-party corroboration of our location when we actually boarded *Last Resort* to take possession.

Vessel Assist's primary purpose is to provide assistance to boaters in distress, most frequently power boaters who run out of gas. In one of those six degrees of separation coincidences, it turns out that the captain of the Vessel Assist boat had been born in the same hospital, the Monmouth Medical Center in Long Branch, New Jersey, about three years after me. We discussed the fact that a famous singer, Bruce Springsteen, had also been born in the same hospital at about the same time. My parent's dearest friend, who was a fixture in my life throughout my childhood, was a gifted author and had a different way of describing the six degrees of separation phenomenon. He said because everywhere he went, somebody knew somebody he knew or was in some other way connected, there must only be 1400 people in the world. He arrived at that number because, as he repeated often, 1400 were all the people he could handle, so since everyone seemed to know someone who was somehow connected to him that must be all the people there are. So whenever I retell a small-world story like this, I always say "I've got a good 1400-people story for you."

Being November, it was a cool, overcast morning in Los Angeles. A recent storm to the north of Los Angeles a few days before had resulted in large residual swells at sea. Arriving at the rendezvous point well ahead of us, Bob decided it was too rough to try to make a transfer, so he sailed farther out. Unfortunately, he didn't immediately advise us what he was doing, so we were more than a little surprised when we arrived at the designated waypoint, only to find no trace of our new boat or Bob. We finally raised him on the VHF radio and received the new latitude and longitude coordinates. Within about 10 minutes we spotted him in the rolling seas and headed in his direction.

Transferring from the small Vessel Assist craft to the larger sailboat was no easy task in the heavy seas, so we had a few hair-raising moments while Sharon and I scampered aboard. Once aboard, there was a fair amount of paperwork to plow through, although we had reviewed everything in advance to ensure there would be no snags during the actual closing of the sale. There was the final contract of sale, an application for documentation by the U.S. Coast Guard, a ship's station license application for the radios on board, and of course, I had to hand over the largest check I'd ever written in my life, since we were paying cash. Once that was done, we had to document the date, so we had brought a copy of the *Los Angeles Times* for that day with us and Bob took our picture holding up the paper. This was the only picture I can remember where Sharon didn't have a smile on her face. She had the most serious case of sticker-shock I've ever seen.

When Bob jumped through mid-air to the pitching deck of the Vessel Assist boat, the reality finally sank in, we owned this boat and I was now the skipper. We decided we would spend a few hours sailing her on our own before we ventured back into port. Normally, we would have been required to leave for Mexico immediately, but there is an exemption to the rules that allows for tolling the time spent in California if it is for the purpose of making

97

repairs. This exemption was designed to benefit the numerous marine supply and repair companies in California who would have lost a lot of business otherwise. Prior to leaving the dock that last morning, we discovered a few additional problems that needed attention. Back at the dock we also discovered that in the rough water the Vessel Assist boat had marred the newly-applied name graphic on the port side, so among the other chores, we had to order a new graphic.

The problems mostly involved things that were loose, but when we started to investigate why the WiFi receiver wasn't working, we discovered that the active USB cables had been installed backwards. I remember in his frustration to try to rectify the problem at the last minute, Bob had damaged one of the cables and we had to leave without a working WiFi system. But all in all, things at that point seemed to be pretty much going as expected. We had been warned on numerous occasions that a newly commissioned boat of this complexity was going to experience a lot of problems before we got everything sorted out. We would soon learn just how prophetic those words would prove to be.

That night we had a small, impromptu christening party aboard *Last Resort* at the dock in Marina del Rey. Norm had gone out of his way to prepare a formal ceremony and I had purchased a pre-scored bottle of champagne wrapped in netting and designed for the purpose. With an assembled audience of a dozen or so people, Norm did a nice job of officiating. I had also prepared a short toast from literature I found on the Internet, which I delivered to the sound of clinking champagne glasses.

When it came time to actually christen the new vessel, the duties fell on Sharon. Positioned on the bow, champagne bottle raised in hand, she leaned over the bow pulpit and prepared to give it a mighty whack against the bow roller. Much to her surprise, instead of the sounds of breaking glass and bubbling champagne, the shock of the seemingly unbreakable bottle colliding with the stainless steel created a resounding thud as it reverberated and careened, unbroken, out of her hand and plopped into the water. We all simultaneously expressed our hope that this wouldn't be a bad

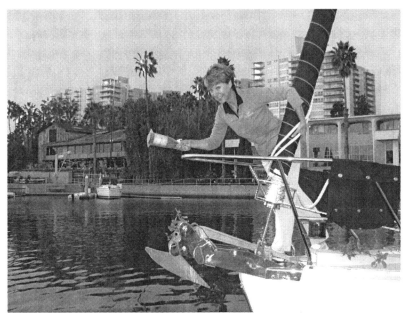

Sharon consigns this unbroken champagne bottle, completely intact, to a watery grave.

omen of some sort. Based on our experiences during the course of the maiden voyage that would follow, it might well have been.

I don't think either of us slept much that night. I was consumed for long hours going over as many systems as possible, refreshing my memory on the stack of manuals I'd read months before and anticipating the cruise ahead, as well as the complexities of the paperwork required to officially enter Mexico. We had planned to depart at a reasonable hour and stop in Newport Harbor, where we were to dine with some friends from the Catalina Fleet #1 group and show off the boat.

The trip started out at 11:30 a.m., slightly delayed while the dealer hurriedly attended to the last few remaining details. We departed in a lovely light breeze and sailed the first third of the trip without the motor. However, when we rounded Point Vicente, as often happens, the wind was blanketed by the land mass of the Palos Verdes peninsula and we had to motor. We had been sailing with the boat in reverse gear to avoid prop cavitation, which creates significant drag, and when I tried to put the shift lever in neutral to start the engine, it wouldn't budge. After repeated tries, the lever came loose. Clearly a cable had been dislodged in the process, because the engine would only shift into reverse or neutral.

After placing an urgent call to Bob, our dealer, I learned that the gears should only be shifted with the engine running, a different procedure than I'd used for years on the Catalina 36. After receiving a thorough explanation of where and how the linkage is connected, Norm and I set out to make the repair. We managed to get the boat into forward gear and we continued on. Uncertain if the repair would hold or if we could put the boat in reverse at the exact moment required to come to a smooth stop in a guest slip, we decided to change our plans and put into Long Beach. Unfortunately, this meant skipping the Newport stop and the chance to see our friends there. The Long Beach Yacht Club has a very long dock in front of the club that would be vacant mid-week at that time of year, assuring us a safe place to land until we could have our makeshift repair professionally checked. I had used the same mechanic for over 15 years, so it was a blessing to me that this problem arose near Long Beach and I promptly contacted Jim to see if he could make an early morning call to double check our work.

Satisfied that the repair was properly done and with a little fine tuning of the adjustment, Jim signed us off and we continued on our way. The second planned stop on our route was Oceanside. There was no wind, so we had to motor the entire 54 miles. We took turns on watch and Norm taught me a lot about the chartplotter, as he had a similar unit on his own boat. We customized all the various display screens to meet our needs and I showed Norm how to plot a route. Norm had never used the routing function, but after he played with it a little he saw the advantages and has started programming routes for most of his trips now, as well.

We still had our faithful Boston Whaler in tow. I noticed early on that towing the Whaler, while running at 3000 rpm to achieve a cruising speed of seven knots, we consumed an inordinate amount of fuel. I was a little upset about that, worrying what our long-range fuel costs might be. Those were the first thoughts I'd had that maybe towing the Boston Whaler for long-range cruising wasn't going to be such a great idea.

Earlier in the year, at the Catalina Rendezvous in July, I had met a couple that had just completed a trip from California to Australia in their own Catalina 470 and I remembered them saying emphatically that we didn't want to be towing the Boston Whaler behind us "like a caboose" when we crossed an ocean. Watching the fuel gauge, the memory of that conversation was brought back to mind.

The Oceanside Yacht Club guest dock was on a first-come, first-served basis. By the time we arrived, the club was closed, but since the dock appeared to be unoccupied, we tied up and after hooking up the water and power, spent a quiet evening aboard. We all enjoyed watching a movie, one of several that Charlene had been good enough to bring along.

We got an early start in the morning, departing at 7:30 a.m. The channel entrance was calm as we departed Oceanside, but Norm told us a chilling story. When they brought their boat back from Mexico almost a decade earlier, they had been caught in a ferocious storm that materialized into something much worse than originally forecast. Finding themselves in 18-foot, dangerous seas, he ignored the orders of the Coast Guard and crossed the bar into Oceanside Harbor. Harbor bar crossings in heavy seas represent high risk and in some conditions all entrance bars need to be closed. So it was, on this day, when Norm was desperately seeking safe harbor for his boat and crew.

Norm went on to say this bar crossing was one of the most harrowing experiences of his sailing career. Apparently the local Harbor Patrol officials were pretty upset that he had disobeyed their warnings not to enter. Norm and Charlene, on the other hand, were just happy to be safe and sound in the harbor, exhausted from fighting the large seas for many hours.

We had an uneventful trip to San Diego and used the time to study and experiment with the numerous functions of the chartplotter. We also tested the MARPA (Mini Automatic Radar Plotting Aid) collision avoidance system included in the radar software. We locked onto a military ship that we thought would make a good target, jokingly hoping they didn't interpret this as a hostile act which would draw their fire. For a long time we didn't think our system was working because the ship didn't appear to be moving. We all had a good laugh when we finally figured out the Navy ship was holding station and actually wasn't moving.

Upon entering the outer channel to the San Diego Harbor, we were hailed by another U.S. Navy warship. The radio operator didn't seem to know port from starboard and it took awhile to sort out the passing instructions so she could pass on our starboard side. "It wasn't much of a warship, but more of a scow," as Norm noted.

We had a hard time securing a reservation for a slip in San Diego in advance of our arrival. It was surprising to us that all of the yacht clubs were full, as were all the marinas we called. We had found ourselves in the middle of boats preparing for the annual southward migration that occurs every fall. We were on the final leg to San Diego when I thought to call my friend Gary at the charter company. Gary pulled a few strings and managed to get us into the Kona Kai Marina. It wasn't cheap at $1.50 a foot, but we were happy just to have a place to put in.

After leaving Marina del Rey, we had tried a few times *en route* to use the Pactor modem to send email, but we couldn't get it to work. It turned out that the guru of Sailmail and the Pactor modem is a fellow named Shea, who hails from San Diego. I was able to reach him on the phone and he agreed to come by the boat. He quickly diagnosed that one of the connections between the computer and the radio was incorrect and that the software needed configuration. He was in a hurry so we didn't do much testing. That night, when I had time to get back to it, I was successful in sending emails through Sailmail. We got a surprise when the radio started transmitting the emails, because most of the electronics on the boat started lighting up or going off. The toilets flushed, the bow thruster came on, all the LED lights on the panel lit up and the stereo crackled. We were excited that we now had the option to access our email almost anywhere in the world through Sailmail's extensive network of linked radio stations, but Norm and I definitely thought it was abnormal for the electronics to all act so oddly.

The next morning we awoke with nervous excitement, anxious to leave San Diego, downbound for sea and heading to the Coral Hotel Marina in Ensenada, Mexico. As we left, we had 100 feet or less of visibility due to dense fog. As soon as we cleared the slip and entered the wide channel, I tried to engage the autopilot. Much to my dismay, it wouldn't engage. After trying repeatedly to engage the malfunctioning autopilot, we had to face the reality of a 62-mile trip without self-steering, meaning one of us would have to be on the helm at all times. The wind never materialized during the entire trip, so Norm and I spent most of our time trouble-shooting the problem and trying, without success, to reach Bob, our dealer, for help. The Globalstar phone, which I had only used once before, refused to lock onto a signal during the entire trip. I also tried sending email to Bob using the single sideband radio and Pactor modem, and while the email seemed to transmit successfully, we never did get a response from Bob and assumed he was unavailable. We had to take turns at the helm. Having the Boston Whaler in tow kept our speed below seven knots, so it took a long 10 hours to reach Ensenada and the entire crew was exhausted by the end of the passage.

It was a good thing for us that Norm had some local knowledge of the Coral Hotel Marina, because when we arrived the channel entrance was completely shrouded in fog with visibility of only a few hundred feet. One thing with which anyone sailing in Mexico must contend is the inaccuracy of the charts. Mexico's charts were all created in the late 1800s and they simply don't match up with the modern GPS chartplotting we employ now. The chart for Ensenada doesn't show the Coral Hotel Marina at all and the shoreline at this location is charted almost 500 yards from the actual location. Maptech and others have compensated by including overlays produced from aerial photography, which improves the accuracy to modern standards. But it's still unnerving to pull into a strange port with restricted visibility.

As tired as I was, when we arrived at the Coral Hotel Marina, it was still imperative to initiate the first round of what Captains Pat and John Rains, in their popular cruising guide, *Mexico Boating Guide*, describe as the "Paperwork Cha, Cha©." The rules regarding initial clearance vary widely from country to country and even within different parts of Mexico. I'd learned this lesson during my cruising days in the Caribbean. As it's sometimes hard to determine what the exact rule is in advance, I always followed the practice of leaving the entire crew on board and striking out alone, passports in hand, to clear in with the local officials. Fortunately for us, Fito's office is a designated agent of the Ensenada Port Captain and they graciously handle the initial port clearance as a service to their guests. So all I had to do that first day was take everyone's passports up to the office, fill out a crew list, pay a $40.00 clearance fee and the marina office took care of the rest.

Since we arrived on a weekend, I normally would have had to leave the next day, a Monday, to go through the entire paperwork process, but because Monday was a holiday, I made an appointment with Fito's office to have their courtesy service driver take me to the appropriate office on Tuesday at 9:00 a.m. to help walk me through the process, translating as needed.

On Sunday morning, Norm and Charlene left very early because they had to get back to organize their upcoming charity function. After they left, I set about reaching the dealer to discuss the autopilot malfunction and doing some routine chores around the boat. It was only then that I would discover the full extent of our troubles. When we first arose, Sharon noticed that the LED lights on the refrigerator control panel weren't illuminated. Later in the morning, Sharon decided to do a load of laundry, only to find that there was no power to the washer-dryer, a compact combination unit mounted in the forward head. After discussing all this during several international phone calls with the dealer, he decided it would be best to bring the boat back to San Diego. I told him it would be quite an effort for just the two of us to make that long trip without the benefit of an operational autopilot, so he agreed to hire a delivery captain to help us.

We discovered several other problems over the weekend, so the list of repairs was growing on a daily basis. Bob had provided us with a home-made series of hoses and filters that we were told to use whenever we hooked up to the municipal water supply in Ensenada. We hadn't done that as of Tuesday morning, so shortly before the time I was scheduled to leave to attend to the various official requirements, I had opened up the compartment under the floorboards where the water tank manifold is located so that I could switch to a full water tank. It was at that moment I noticed water in the battery compartments, dangerously close to topping the batteries and shorting out our electrical system. Unfortunately, this repair couldn't wait, so I dove into it, knowing I was going to miss my scheduled appointment.

We had noticed a water leak during the pre-delivery process, but when we mentioned it to the rigger; he just shrugged his shoulders and said "All boats leak." This wasn't a satisfactory answer, but with time short and the leaks seemingly minor, we had decided we'd worry about it at a later date. After a thorough investigation, I finally isolated the problem. It turns out there is an elbow joint attached to one of the water lines on the water heater. It became obvious what the problem was when I determined the fitting was not securely screwed into the socket. To do so, one needed to remove the cover on the water heater's electrical panel. My guess was that the plumbers at the factory were not authorized to remove the electrical panel, so rather than properly tightening the fitting, they simply applied an excess of joint filler, a temporary solution at best. Since we'd heard of this problem on other C470s, we dutifully reported it to Gerry at Catalina Yachts. We were rewarded with a "thank you" and a comment that they were changing the installation procedure to avoid this problem in the future. By the time I finished making this repair and pumping all the water out of the battery compartment, I had missed my appointment and had to reschedule.

When I went to Fito's office for the rescheduled afternoon appointment, I was introduced to a very pleasant young fellow who was assigned to assist me with the task ahead. We drove a couple of miles to a nice, clean building near the main Ensenada Harbor. I was about to experience the Mexican "Paperwork Cha, Cha" first hand. One thing I learned in the Caribbean was that you have to maintain an abundance of patience and humility when dealing with port authorities. It doesn't hurt to have a sense of humor either. I was particularly bemused by the process in Mexico.

Due to widespread corruption, the government doesn't trust the bureaucrats in the numerous offices that you must visit to handle money. After each visit, whether to the Port Captain, immigration, customs or fishing permit office, you have to go next to the bank, which thankfully maintains an office within the same building, make your payment and obtain a receipt. You then return to the office you last visited, present the receipt and obtain the appropriate stamps or papers. I have been told that before this office was built, the clearance process could take all day because the various offices were spread out all over town.

Since Fito had already handled the port clearance paperwork, I was able to skip the preliminary visit to the Port Captain's office, so my knowledgeable driver took me first to the line for the Immigration Office (*Migración*). There I filled out the application for our tourist cards and presented our passports. After they were reviewed, I was handed a form and pointed in the direction of the bank office across the building. This was my first visit to the bank. The clerk spoke no English, but smiled affably and happily took my money. Once back at *Migración* I quickly completed the process and moved on to the Customs Office (*Audana*).

Aduana is where you obtain a Temporary (10-year) Import Permit for the boat and all her equipment and also where you push the button to see if you get the green or red light. A red light means you can expect a visit from an armed contingent of inspectors. I'm told about five percent of the time some poor sailor gets the red light. I was lucky and breathed a small sigh of relief when the green light illuminated brightly. Then it was back to see my new-found buddy at the bank. I joked that we "had to stop meeting like this," which my driver translated to some appreciative laughter.

I managed to skip the line at the office where the fishing licenses are issued (*Commisión Nacional de Acuacultura y Pesca, Oficina de Pesca*). In an effort to reduce the complexity of the process in Ensenada, Sharon and I had attended to this task ahead of time at a sporting goods store in San Diego. In Mexico, if you have so much as a fish hook or a small scrap of fishing line aboard ship, everyone must have a fishing license. The fines are steep and can even

106

include confiscation of your boat, so while we've never actually heard of it happening, we surely weren't about to take any chances.

On the way back to the marina I thanked my driver for his assistance and gave him a $10.00 tip. I'll never forget his grateful comment that "Now I can feed my family tonight." There is a serious dichotomy between the wealth of the few ruling families in Mexico and the general population, and while it is slowly improving, the average worker in Mexico is still grossly underpaid. Until Mexico achieves parity and solves some of the corruption problems that plague its government at all levels, I don't see how they can emerge from third-world status.

Without a functioning autopilot, we wouldn't be doing much sailing during the balance of that first week in Mexico. But since I needed all the docking practice I could get, we did manage a couple of day sails later in the week after the fog moved out for good. During those sails we explored the main harbor of Ensenada and ventured out to Islas Todos Santos to investigate the anchorage possibilities. We had read and heard conflicting reports about the difficulties presented by the existence of an aqua-farming operation there. It looked like we would be able to anchor without difficulty, so we decided to make an overnight stay on a future visit.

Reluctantly, at the end of the following weekend we had to leave the boat and head back to Scottsdale to attend to mail and other matters that needed our attention. We were a little unhappy to be leaving the boat, but security at the Coral Hotel Marina was excellent. We had tipped one of the night watchmen generously and he had promised to keep an extra close eye on our boat. As the months went on, we made good friends with all the staff at the marina and we never worried about security.

Not wanting to repeat our experience at the Tijuana border crossing, where we had experienced long delays during our previous trip to position the cars, we obtained some directions from Fito and headed off to Tecaté *en route* to Scottsdale. This route took us through the local vineyards and we were treated to a delightful scenic drive through wine country, followed by some fairly significant mountain roads. We would be pleasantly rewarded when we only had to wait five minutes in line before being greeted by the

107

U.S. Customs officer at the border. It's a nice drive going that way too, because even the badlands and sand dunes near El Centro are quite scenic. We would repeat this trip on numerous occasions during our seven-month stay in Mexico, using the time to listen to recorded Spanish language lessons. On one trip we tried another route, continuing further east while still in Mexico intending to cross the border at Mexicali. It turned out to take much longer, primarily due to the need to travel 10 miles of narrow, winding road carved precariously into a steep, sheer mountain. The mountainside was littered with hundreds of car carcasses that must have once belonged to travelers like ourselves, convincing us never to take this route again.

Because we were still monitoring my health very closely, and as Sharon was in the process of actively building her new business, our practice was to spend two or three weeks on the boat, punctuated by a couple of weeks back in Scottsdale. Communications aboard ship were only marginal at the Coral Hotel Marina. The WiFi Internet connection was slow and undependable. Therefore, the Vonage phones only worked sporadically and we'd often find ourselves without Internet access. Single sideband radio communications were blocked by the mountains that surround Ensenada and the Globalstar phone refused to work. After doing some online research, I learned that Globalstar was having a lot of problems with their satellites and I decided to swap out the Globalstar phone for an Iridium model. While the Iridium phone and air time costs were significantly higher, the Iridium network was extremely reliable and would work virtually anywhere we planned to sail.

We both remember our time in Mexico with fondness. We met some wonderful people and loved the friendly, warm grace of the Mexican people. One character I will always remember is Chilly Willie. His real name was Miguel, but since it seemed that half of Mexican men are named Miguel, this fellow picked "Chilly Willie" as his nickname so he would stand out. Chilly Willie worked for the American owner of one of the fishing boats on the dock and every morning he'd greet me with a smile and an *hola* before he set about his daily routine of polishing and shining. Chilly Willie was quick-witted and was always making wise cracks or pulling practical jokes on me. But he was a qualified skipper and an accomplished fisherman, as I would learn on several fishing trips we took together. For a poor people, Mexicans are an unusually generous lot and Chilly Willie was no different. I had once purchased a case of Gatorade in Mexico, only to learn that they actually manufacture a much spicier version for that market. As it didn't agree with my hyper-sensitive stomach, I gave Chilly Willie the whole case. I learned later that he only kept a few bottles for himself and his wife, distributing the rest to the dock hands and marina workers.

In December, under the able command of Captain Mark, whom the dealer had hired for the purpose, we sailed the boat back to San Diego for repairs. Mark had brought along a new, dealer-supplied replacement computer for the autopilot, so fortunately we didn't have to hand-steer all the way back to San Diego. Once there, Bob had dispatched a small army of people to work on our problems, including Byron, a highly qualified rigger who we have grown to respect and made an honorary member of our family. It was a good thing too, because just as we arrived in San Diego our Freedom 25 inverter-charger started overheating, turning itself off automatically. It would have to be replaced while in port.

Overall the trip to San Diego was highly successful, and with the exception of the washer-dryer which had to be removed from the boat and delivered to Ventura, California for repairs, everything else was fixed in short order. After all the problems we'd experienced, this was a big relief to us.

We were using a standard DirecTV 3-LMN satellite dish with a rigid stern mount to watch standard and high definition U.S. television programming. We discovered in Mexico that because of the frequent surge in the Coral Hotel Marina, we couldn't tie the boat down tight enough for the satellite dish to maintain a steady lock on the signal, so television reception had been impossible. Rather than spending more than $5,000.00 at the time for a gyro-stabilized system, I opted to install a much cheaper FollowMeTV© system while we were in San Diego. This dish mount is two dimensional, tracking the compass heading of the satellite as the boat moves. It wasn't designed to work in any kind of seaway or rough anchorage, but it performed exceptionally well once we got back to

Mexico and enabled us to enjoy the extensive menu of DirecTV programming while there, even with the constant shifting of the boat's position when the surge was running.

The return voyage was very pleasant. Catalina again authorized us to use Mark's services as captain so we wouldn't be alone on the trip back to Mexico. While *en route* we had picked up a Coast Guard pan-pan warning that there would be 15-to-20 foot swells near the Channel Islands, so we were all grateful we weren't sailing in those waters. Once we arrived back at the Coral Hotel Marina we broke out the Scotch and Mark and Sharon toasted our safe arrival and completion of a successful trip. Sharon and I didn't know that this celebration would turn out to be premature, for our problems were far from over.

As we gained more confidence with each subsequent day sail, we started to venture farther and farther from port. We were finally ready to attempt our first overnight anchorage at Islas Todos Santos. Upon our arrival we found that a large powerboat was anchored inside the only cove that looked suitable for anchoring. Since the seas were calm and the forecast called for fair weather, we opted to anchor in deeper water just outside the cove. We had 200 feet of chain aboard at that time and had to use all of it at this spot. There was an additional 200 feet of nylon rode attached to the chain that we could have deployed, but the transition from chain to rode on the windlass is tricky and I opted not to risk it. As we were anchoring, the fellow who tends the aqua-farm operation came over in his *panga* as a courtesy to indicate where the mooring lines for the large pens led, making sure we avoided them with our anchor.

Once satisfied we were secure, we decided to hop in the Boston Whaler, which we had towed along, to explore the various coves and perhaps visit with the folks on the large powerboat. As we came into the inner cove, they appeared on deck and started frantically signaling something and gesturing for us to be careful. We soon discovered that one of the huge mooring lines for the aqua-farm stretched across the entire entrance to the inner cove at far too shallow a depth for us to have made it across in our sailboat with her eight-foot draft. Lucky for us we hadn't ventured in. After an

110

enjoyable visit with wine and hors d'oeuvres aboard their boat, we headed back to *Last Resort.*

It was winter, so the days were short and the nights cool. Once we were settled in below, I decided to use the radar to keep an anchor watch, setting an alarm ring at just the right distance from the boat to warn us if we should drag anchor and start drifting towards the shore. The winds had kicked up with occasional gusts as high as 25 knots, so I set up the plasma TV to display the radar screen to keep a visual fix until I was sure our anchor would hold. Around 11:00 p.m., while we were relaxing and reading, the radar anchor alarm went off. When I looked at the radar screen, I was amazed to see a huge blob heading right for us at high speed. I sprang up on deck just in time to see our friends on the power boat, which dwarfed our 47 feet, speed dangerously close as they made a hasty retreat from the cove.

Somewhat displeased, I waited until they cleared the aqua-farms and raised them on the VHF radio to find out what had happened. It turned out that their anchors had both dragged and they were barely able to hoist the main anchor aboard before they would have drifted into the dangerous, jagged rocks ashore. In fact, they had to abandon their stern anchor in their haste, only being able to hurriedly affix a large fender to it as they retreated. They asked us if we would mind retrieving the anchor and bringing it back the next day when we returned, suggesting there was an "expensive bottle of champagne" in it for us. We would have done that for them anyway, but the offer of champagne sounded pretty good to Sharon.

The next morning Sharon and I took the Whaler and went exploring, sticking our nose into every little nook and cranny we could find. We never found a decent beach on which to land the Whaler, so after we had seen what we could from the water, we went into the cove to retrieve the powerboat's stern anchor. Their stern anchor was almost as big as our CQR 44-pound primary anchor and we struggled to get the whole rig, anchor, chain and rode, aboard the Boston Whaler.

When we saw how difficult it was to find a suitable location to beach the Whaler that was pretty much the final straw for her. We made up our minds that we were going to have to dispatch with the Whaler and get a dinghy suitable for beach landings. I resolved that I would start researching what might work best for our needs as soon as we got back to port and had Internet access.

After securing our boat back at the Coral Hotel Marina, we jumped in the Whaler to return the anchor. Remembering our struggle to wrestle the thing aboard for them, we rather expected the couple to invite us over for a chat or perhaps to make plans to get together for dinner at the restaurant. Instead, only the husband appeared on the stern to receive his recovered anchor. Having never left our dinghy and as we got ready to push off, he thrust a paper bag with a bottle inside in an almost off-hand manner. When we returned to *Last Resort*, we found that instead of champagne, the bag contained a bottle of cheap white wine. We would have actually felt better to have just received a thank you, rather than an off-handed 'payment' for our efforts. Many of our friends are power boaters and I hate to perpetuate the prejudice that some sailors have for power boaters, but sometimes it's warranted and I thought this was one of those times.

Before we left Ensenada, I had researched the various dinghy options and settled on an 11-foot Advanced Cat with a 15-horse-power Mercury engine. I was spoiled by the Boston Whaler, and while I had lost all the excess weight I carried before I was diagnosed with cancer and was getting quite sure-footed again, I wasn't ready to sacrifice the stability of the Whaler. The design of this new catamaran was wider than a standard dinghy, therefore providing stability and also increasing the cargo and passenger capacity. When we got back to Scottsdale, we immediately ordered the new dinghy and anxiously awaited the arrival of the boxes. It was just before Christmas and we decided this would have to suffice as our Christmas present to ourselves, because it was fairly expensive. Sharon joked that it wasn't quite as attractive on her as, say, a new dress or a piece of jewelry. When it arrived, I couldn't wait to open the box and inflate the dinghy, so we dragged all 115 pounds of it into our family room and inflated it until it seemed to fill almost half the family room.

We were both anticipating our next trip to Ensenada, not only because we couldn't wait to try out the dinghy, but because Sharon's daughter, Roxanne, and her fiancé, Ingo, were planning a visit. Roxanne had followed her heart and moved to Stuttgart, Germany not long before, to be with Ingo and take a job with Daimler-Chrysler, where Ingo also worked.

We were in for a surprise when we tried to deflate the dinghy and get it into the car. It just barely fit and I had to enlist the aid of Pablo, the neighborhood gardener and his assistant, to help me push, pull, stuff and finally cram the thing into the back seat. We were also laden down with Christmas gifts for the kids. Sharon had gone all out in anticipation of their visit. As we approached the border in San Diego we both nervously prayed that when we pushed the button the light would be green. Once again, our luck prevailed and we sailed through. Had we been inspected, there would have been a hefty duty to pay on the dinghy. While I might have been able to convince them it was covered by the Temporary (10-year) Import Permit, I hadn't thought to bring it with me.

When we arrived in Mexico, I could barely wait to inflate the new dinghy, mount the motor and take it out for a spin. With the help of a couple of my local friends, we managed to get it all organized and took it out for a joy ride. Because the motor was new, we had to break it in before we could really open it up, so that would come later. Once back at the slip, we hoisted the dinghy onto the foredeck, where we had planned to store it. I had the old, wooden motor mount that I had used aboard the Catalina 36, but I discovered it wouldn't fit the stern-rail configuration on the new boat, so I had purchased a plastic one that looked like it would be easier to modify. Once I had it in place, we hoisted the new outboard motor aboard. This 15-horsepower Mercury motor weighs about 85 pounds and it looked to me like the flimsy motor mount I had purchased wouldn't hold in a seaway with any pounding or shock loading, so I set about researching a better solution and later ordered a sturdier mount.

We had a great time with Roxanne and Ingo, but not without some excitement. Soon after they arrived we took them out for a great afternoon sail in brisk wind. Ingo took to the sailing like a duck to water, although I don't think Roxanne really cares much for it. Their second or third night aboard there were severe Santa Ana winds, those warm winds that blow off the California and Arizona deserts, creating havoc in the fire-prone hills of Southern California and making the north-facing anchorages of the Channel Islands and Catalina extremely dangerous to boaters. We were heeling over pretty dramatically in the slip and clocking winds close to 40 knots, or more than 45 miles per hour. Everyone was pretty excited by this, watching the anemometer and calling out the wind speed like an announcer at Pimlico. We divided our time that evening between shouting out wind speeds of 25, then 30, then 35-knots, and so on, and watching a movie on DVD.

When Christmas day arrived, the weather was spectacular, one of those days that accounts for the huge westward migration of weather-weary Easterners to Southern California every year. We had an enjoyable morning sitting outside in the cockpit where we opened all the gifts and Sharon served brunch. I remember one of my gifts from Sharon was a calendar of exotic islands around the world. I was somewhat surprised when I realized I had visited six of the twelve islands showcased in the calendar.

That afternoon there was a pot luck Christmas dinner organized by the local cruisers net that convened on the VHF radio every morning at 8:00 a.m. So when we finished opening and enjoying our Christmas presents, Sharon packed up some snacks and we headed off to Cruiseport Marina in the main Ensenada harbor, the location of the party. When we arrived, someone told us that the *Black Pearl*, from the movie *Pirates of the Caribbean*, was moored there, so we set off, camera in hand, to check it out. We got some good shots and enjoyed looking all around this replica. I was impressed by the huge size of the boat and the attention to detail. That was the highlight of the afternoon, although the gift exchange proved to be a lot of fun as well.

It was during this trip that the four of us set off to explore La Bufadora, located about 15 miles southwest of Ensenada at Punta Banda. Sharon is an excellent writer and always manages to present the whimsical side of our travels and adventures. It would be no different for our trip to *La Bufadora*, which she described in a short article she wrote for our website, as follows:

La Bufadora.... A non-speaker of Spanish might wonder what that is — some low-lidded, throaty lounge singer who's seen better days? Perhaps a shard of Mayan crockery inlaid with some sort of buffalo-like beast? No, it's an ocean blowhole on Punta Banda, just south of the Baja California, Mexico seaside town of Ensenada.

The Spanish verb *bufar* means "to snort" and snort it does, with plumes of seawater shooting through rocks, spurting 60-to-70 feet into the air. They're not bluffing, there's plenty of puffing.

And that goes for the street vendors, too. They're the best part of the show. Aggressive, but harmless, they're like a church carnival on steroids. I look at a pair of sunglasses emblazoned with a giant, bejeweled "D" being offered for $10.00. I walk away and the price drops to $7.00. I now own a lovely pair of "name-brand" shades. We continue making our way through the gauntlet of eager hawkers touting jewelry, stained glass, serapes, wood carvings and the inevitable sombrero or two for almost a quarter of a mile.

My husband, the expert, advises me to not make eye contact and keep moving. I drive forward in a determined fashion, like we're heading for the fountain of youth. (Well, I admit I did linger a little bit around the food stands. They were selling hollowed-out coconuts stuffed with something that must have been delectable judging from the lines of hungry-looking people.)

Finally, we reach the stone balustrade jutting out over the edge of a 50-foot cliff. The rocky coastline, 70-degree weather, turquoise waters, bluer-than-blue skies – it's hard to believe it's the middle of winter and parts of the Midwest, New Mexico and Colorado are having record snowstorms.

The crowd at La Bufadora reminds me of first-time viewers of the Grand Canyon: Seeing the power of nature displayed so vividly makes you go, "Ah!" We gaze and gasp at the impressive power of the ocean trying to defy gravity. We linger for a full round of family photos – me with the hubster; my daughter with her fiancé, etc. – before we continue to the day's final highlight, lunch at a seaside restaurant with an incredible ocean view. I am bedazzled, despite my new sunglasses.

We drove back to Scottsdale shortly after New Year's. We would return to Mexico at least once a month. Each time, we would sail farther and we were slowly gaining confidence in our new boat, and more importantly, in our own ability to handle her. Finally, by March, we had gained enough confidence to embark alone on our first overnight cruise south of Punta Banda. We knew that once we rounded Punta Banda and headed south, we would truly be on our own. There would be no Vessel Assist or friendly U.S. Coast Guard to help us if we got in trouble. It was near the end of March when we set off for Puerto Santo Tomas, a sleepy little fishing village located 23 nautical miles south of Ensenada.

At last we were finally able to take a real cruise out of the Hotel Coral Marina. We had a delightful sail to this really tiny fishing village, where there are less than 15 tiny cottages lining the coast. On the road leading to the point is a peach-colored arch worthy of a Ben Hur movie, with the name Puerto Santo Tomas emblazoned over the road and more tiny cottages behind it. In the bay below town a dozen modest *pangas* painted in bright pastels were moored.

Two familial groups were gathering mussels from the stony shore. They paused for the amusement we provided as I threaded *Last Resort* this way and that to avoid maze-like clumps of seaweed. We dropped her anchor once, twice, well…three times, until I was happy with the final location. Even if it took 40 tries, I knew neither of us would have slept until I got it right. We were tucked safe and sound in our cozy anchorage, and calmly, as we had our brand new flopper stopper out. Unfortunately, we would later lose this ingenious device due to a faulty snap shackle. I felt particularly badly because this had been a gift from Bob, our Catalina dealer. I hated to tell him of our loss, but he was so gracious, he later replaced it, so that made two nice gifts he'd given us.

116

So here we were, relaxed at last, when we heard….nothing. That's not good. We should have been hearing our generator cranking out power. Seaweed had clogged its intake valve. After unloading what seemed like a ton of stuff out of a three-by-four-foot storage space underneath the Pullman berth, I replaced it with my sweaty, cursing self. The whole evening passed in a blur as I grunted and groaned while attacking the problem. Once I was able to clear out the blockage, we settled down to watch *American Idol* in our warm, diesel-heated cabin. The anchorage was amazingly calm, so the FollowMeTV satellite dish mount was able to provide us with a surprisingly consistent picture.

A sunny morning found no mussel-gatherers on the beach. It occurred to me there had been no lights in the little village the night before. There was no electricity in town. We suffered some pangs of guilt as we realized we had more electricity on our boat last night than the entire town, thanks to our generator.

We had a terrific return sail in 18-to-20-knot winds. *Last Resort* handled the upwind sail beautifully, despite facing some big seas,

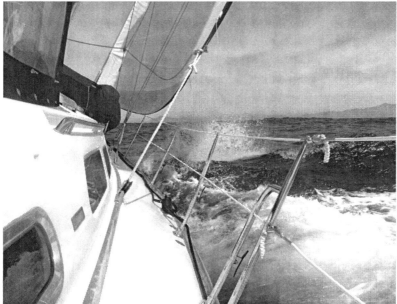

Last Resort close-hauled off coast of Baja, California.

sometimes up to 8-to-10-feet. We ducked back into our home port as the sun began to set. There was a lovely full moon and the beginning of a Santa Ana wind that promised warm temperatures the next day. It was taking some time, but we were becoming more and more accustomed to the cruising life.

It was a life, it seemed, prone to a never-ending cycle of equipment failures and constant repairs. Back in Ensenada after another intervening trip to Scottsdale, we were preparing to go out for a lovely afternoon of sailing. As I was performing my routine checks, I noticed a serious problem. The goose-neck bracket that attaches the boom to the mast was pulling loose. One of six bolts was completely free of the mast and all the others were dangerously loose. If the boom had separated from the mast in the strong winds we encountered on our return cruise from Puerto Santo Tomas a few weeks earlier, not only would we have been facing a difficult situation, but one of us could have been seriously injured. We had been extremely lucky. The first thing I did was piece together all the hose clamps I could find to secure the fitting to the mast. We obviously weren't going sailing that day, but even in the slip, the force of the surge or a strong wind could have exerted enough pressure to break the boom loose. I wasn't taking any chances.

When I reached Bob to explain the problem, he became very concerned. He thought that the boat should immediately be returned to the United States for repairs and this time he didn't want us aboard, so he arranged for Mark to pick up the boat and return it to Marina del Rey where Bob had the resources to deal with a problem of this magnitude. While the California tax rules allowed us to toll our time while performing legitimate repairs, this trip meant that several weeks would have to be added to our stay in Mexico. We would miss a few of the summer cruises with our yacht clubs that we had been looking forward to, but there was nothing to be done for it. We decided that we would take advantage of the trip to accomplish some other things as well. We had postponed adding air conditioning units in the main salon and the aft stateroom, but it was starting to get warm and it seemed like a good time to do it. Another problem we'd identified was that negotiating the foredeck with the dinghy aboard was cumbersome and created a safety issue. It would be hard to scamper forward in the event the anchor had to be deployed in an emergency or if something else requiring immediate access to the foredeck should occur. The solution was to add davits to the stern of the boat, where we could mount and carry the dinghy, freeing up the foredeck. There was a sacrifice here, because the stern ladder would no longer be available for use as long as the dinghy was hoisted, but on the other hand, it would be so easily accessible that it could double as a life raft. So once all this was organized and the boat moved to Marina del Rey, we hopped in the car and drove ourselves to Los Angeles.

We spent the next month supervising the work. The boom problem was caused by the failure of the boatyard to properly affix the backing plate so that the gooseneck fitting was only held by the aluminum mast, not the reinforcing stainless steel plate into which it should have been fastened. Installing the two air conditioning units was a big undertaking, as was the davit installation. Once all this work was completed, including re-installing the now-repaired washer-dryer, Mark was again retained by Catalina Yachts to return the boat to Mexico.

Ever since we sailed the boat to Mexico, Norm had been discussing the possibility of joining us for a cruise to Turtle Bay. This is a convenient stopping-point for southbound cruisers heading into Mexico, located just about half-way down the west coast of Baja, and Norm had been there once before when he'd crewed in the Baja Ha-Ha. The Baja Ha-Ha is an informal race and rally for almost 200 boats that make the annual fall migration to Mexico for the winter sailing season. Since we had agreed to the trip, I had stocked up on five-gallon plastic fuel jugs at the local Home Depot store in Scottsdale and we had a car full of a dozen of them on this trip to the boat. Yet again our luck held and we breezed through the border check point when the green light illuminated.

We decided that since we were going to be taking a long cruise, stopping in mostly uninhabited roadside anchorages *en route* to Turtle Bay, we should get one more practice cruise under our belts. We decided to head back to Puerto Santo Tomas. We had only spent one night there, never venturing ashore. Now that we had our new dinghy and could feasibly make a beach or rock landing, we were anxious to explore this place further.

We had a great sail down, close reaching to Punta Banda and then running before the wind all the way to Puerto Santo Tomas. This time, having already had the experience, I was able to drop the anchor in just the right spot, securing it well in the sand and sea-weed bottom on the first try. We had an extremely relaxing weekend. I had a chance to really test the new dinghy and its capa-bilities and we managed to land it at the decaying boat ramp, where a couple of local fishermen helped us secure the dinghy so we could explore the little village. Now clear of the blocking moun-tains of Ensenada, I was able to practice my radio and email skills with the Pactor modem. After a pleasant return sail in light winds and 75° F. temperature, we finished this last shakedown cruise and returned to Scottsdale to attend to some business before the long trip to Turtle Bay.

The round trip from Ensenada to Turtle Bay is about 575 miles. Given the distance, we had agreed that we would need two weeks to accomplish the voyage. Our departure from the Coral Hotel Marina was delayed for several hours due to the Mexican bureau-cracy. Unlike my first experience, what should have been a simple trip to pick up fishing licenses for Norm and Charlene turned out to be anything but. Norm and I left early so we would arrive just as the offices opened. In true Mexican fashion, the fellow who runs the *Oficina de Pesca* didn't arrive until after 9:15 a.m. Then it turned out the banking office's computers were down, so they couldn't accept payment. Not wanting to lose our parking spot, we had to walk up a large hill to the nearest bank, about a mile away, and then go back with proof of payment and stand in line again to get the licenses stamped.

After posing aboard *Last Resort* for a group shot, we were finally underway a little after 11:00 a.m. Our first stop was Puerto Santo Tomas, with which we were by now well familiar. But this time, we found the anchorage seaweed-laden, so we had to anchor in deeper, rougher water outside the seaweed line in 45 feet. The evening was spent stowing provisions. We were careful to ensure that cans of chicken were kept accessible. Ten years earlier, when

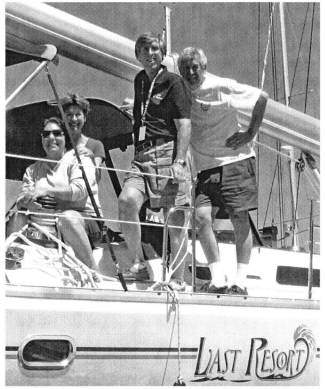

Captain and crew before setting sail downbound for Turtle Bay.

Norm had crewed for a boat during the Baja Ha-Ha, he had come away greatly impressed by the abundance of fresh fish delivered to their stern each evening by fishermen returning home. His crew had found the Baja fishermen so sated with fish that they enjoyed swapping their catch for tins of chicken breast. So we were prepared to barter.

We weighed anchor at approximately 1:10 a.m. so that it would be daylight when we arrived at our destination. We were motoring nicely at seven knots. First light was visible at 4:30 a.m. after we enjoyed a lovely half-moon from the time we departed until daybreak, when it was still visible. We also saw phosphorescence-emitting plankton in the water shortly after departing Puerto Santo Tomas. Watch change started at 5:00 a.m.

when Charlene woke up and relieved Norm. Sharon was up an hour later to relieve me.

As the day wore on, there was no wind and the seas were flat. Charlene and Sharon stood watch as we motored, reading and taking turns snoozing. The air was fresh and cool, but not chilling. Off the coast of Cabo San Quintin, thick fog loomed in the distance. As we arrived, it burned off for the most part. We chugged forward, sliding over silky-smooth, undulating water to sneak between Isla de San Martin and the mainland. We'd been told there is a fishing village on Isla de San Martin, in Hassler's Cove, but we didn't get close enough to really see it. We were intent on avoiding Ben's Rock, a partially submerged rock which breaks in heavy seas, and was the site of the shipwreck of a 100-foot fishing vessel.

We reached Isla San Jeronimo, a rock, noisy with a seal rookery and odorous with sea bird guano, at 5:45 p.m., just in time for dinner. We saw seven whales on our approach — both California gray whales and humpbacks. At one point we passed closely to two grays. One sounded after flashing its tail and the other just roiled like a serpent. Sharon got up at about 1:00 a.m. and went on deck, only to be startled when a whale surfaced not 30 feet from the boat. She watched, in awe, as the water from the whale's blowhole dissipated into the ethereal fog.

We departed at a little after 4:00 a.m., as scheduled, easing *Last Resort* past the potentially engulfing seaweed patches. The scene was eerie as we crossed over flat, fog-wrapped Bahia Sebastian Vizcaino. The wind came up about 15 miles from Cedros Island. We started sailing in about 10 knots and it built to over 20 knots as we approached the north end of the island. When we got very close to the island the fog gradually rolled back and almost biblically, *Isla Cedros* emerged, looking like a Japanese brush painting.

When we rounded into the lee of the island the wind dropped abruptly to zero and we anchored, on the second try, in 30 feet of water with poor holding. Despite that, Norm said it was like being in a slip and that was pretty accurate, as there was virtually no movement. The North Anchorage was dense with raucous and randy elephant seals. That evening we watched as couples would first spar with one another in a process that could only be described

122

as necking and then collapse for 15-minute-long snoozes before facing off with one another again. We greatly enjoyed this setting that was so devoid of people. This must be what Catalina Island was like before we humans arrived.

We saw barely a soul during the four-day journey down Baja's rocky coast. Peopled by fishing communities, tiny pueblos appeared with infrequency. Norm's hankering for fresh fish would apparently have to wait as we had seen no fishing activity.

We had a cool, foggy motor-sail for the rest of the trip. When a little bit of wind did come up, Norm was in the shower and advised that the shower definitely won't drain on a starboard tack. Charlene took her second-ever underway shower too, and that's after several decades of sailing experience.

Once we reached Turtle Bay, or Bahia de Tortugas, the fog cleared completely and we peeled off our caps and foul weather gear in what had quickly become tropically warm, sunny weather. This would be the first time I put the air conditioning units to work. We spent several pleasant days exploring the small town, Puerto San Bartolome (population less than 1,000). We were certain we could find fish for Norm here. After all, Turtle Bay boasts three restaurants. But no, they were all closed for the whole week in honor of Mother's Day. Small familial groups were gathered on their porches awaiting the evening, when there was to be a women-only party to celebrate the holiday.

The local gas concession is run by the Gordo family. Not only was Enrique, one of Gordo's sons, taking care of our fuel needs, but Sharon had already bonded with the whole Gordo family and rumor had it that Sharon and Dolores (Enrique's sister) were seen dancing to the salsa at the bar while I stayed aboard to attend to ship's business.

We were in shock to learn after filling the tanks that we had only needed 45 gallons of fuel after the whole trip down, almost all of which was motoring. Our average speed ended up at 7.23 knots, but we knew that average would get shot to hell on the way back. We had our 12 jerry jugs on the rail, plus one additional jug stored below filled with diesel, so we had 158 gallons of fuel for the return trip.

Our second day in Turtle Bay we ran out of water. We switched to our largest, 62-gallon tank intending to use it for the first time, only to discover no water would come out of it. I had forgotten to switch the heads to salt water and as a result we had unnecessarily used fresh water when flushing the toilets. Because it was a daunting job to get to the tank that wasn't working, requiring removing all the furniture, the air conditioning and heating units with all their pumps and vents, as well as the floor and sub-floor on the port side of the main salon, it was an easy decision to engage Enrique to deliver 150 gallons of water. We knew we couldn't drink this water and that we'd have to shock the whole system with chlorine later, but Norm had thought ahead, so we had at least five gallons of drinking water aboard, enough for the return trip if we conserved.

I discovered on this trip that Sailmail has a service called Shadowmail where they forward only the headers from your regular email account and then you can decide what to download. I was anxious to go to the local Internet Café to clear out my old emails and spam so I could then try out Shadowmail with the single sideband radio without wasting air time downloading spam.

We planned on staying in Turtle Bay until Saturday when we would head back. Our planned route was to go to Islas San Benito, then to San Quintin, Punta Colnett and on into Ensenada. Our strategy would be to depart each port between 1:00 a.m. and 4:00 a.m., motoring as much as we could, assuming the winds calmed down overnight, and then sailing the rest of the day, never getting into any port after dark. We ended up under some time pressure because Norm and Charlene had a charitable event for which they were responsible coming up the next weekend. By now, we had a need to return as well, so we didn't have much time to delay.

One thing that was beginning to baffle me was the weather forecast. There were a handful of sailboats in Turtle Bay, all of whom said they were waiting out forecasted 35-knot winds. On the other hand, I had downloaded a current GRIB file every day and I didn't see any 35-knot winds forecast at all, 15-to-20 being the highest forecast. So I was at a little bit of a loss. GRIB files are tremendously more compact than regular weather charts and because of their size are very well suited for download via wireless means. We had also paid for a commercial forecast from one of several companies that provide this service. This was my first experience with any of the commercial routing and forecasting services, but after the first day, their forecasts proved to be pretty unreliable, making me skeptical of their accuracy.

Nevertheless, we broke a cardinal rule of sailing. We were on a schedule. For the following several days we paid the price, our hull pounding into choppy eight-to-10-foot seas that set our teeth on edge. We had hoped to slide past West Benito Island to the outer waters in order to get the optimum sailing angle on the wind. But the wind turned to near-gale force, coming from the prevailing north-northwest direction. With our hull pounding into each wave, we labored for more than an hour into 25-to-30 knots of wind, occasionally gusting to 35, right on our nose. With an exhausted and apprehensive crew, we decided to alter our course and head for shelter in the lee of *Isla Cedros*. That theory proved to be erroneous and we continued to battle consistent 30-plus knot winds and steep eight-to-10-foot seas breaking over the bow for the duration of the night. Charlene, it turned out, was prone to seasickness in heavy seas, so the poor woman stayed out in the cockpit all night. At times the seas breaking over the boat would fill the cockpit and douse a stoic Charlene.

We eventually put into the North Cedros anchorage at dawn, giving the weary crew a chance at some much-needed rest, although on this occasion, the wind continued to blow with gusts over 30 knots. We were grateful to be in such a solid, seaworthy boat as the winds funneled around the eastern side of Cedros Island.

We spent the rest of the day recovering. We rested and watched cavorting baby seals, who ventured close to check out *Last Resort*. The crew had just sat down to an early supper when the wind shifted and our anchor lost its hold. I started the motor and took the wheel as the crew wolfed down their meals and pulled on their foulies. As we were resetting the anchor, I spotted another sailboat,

Mystic Traveler, making its way upwind through the channel. I hailed them on the VHF radio and talked to the boat's delivery captain who said they left Turtle Bay at 5:00 p.m. and planned to tack northwest after passing north of Cedros, then head straight for San Diego.

Once we secured the anchor, the crew rested until 3:00 a.m. Sharon volunteered to stand anchor watch because she is the only one who had the ability to actually sleep once we got underway. She said she played solitaire, paced back and forth and listened to music in an effort to stay awake. The wind died down considerably by the middle of the night and the next day we made great early-morning progress motor-sailing north with just a reefed mainsail set. Eventually, we were amazed to find that we had almost caught up with *Mystic Traveler*. They had been hard-pressed by wind, waves and current and struggled all night long for very little northward progress. We were wise to wait it out.

We continued on into winds that once again built to 25-to-30 knots. We did enjoy a much-appreciated lift forecast by our weather service when the wind shifted westerly and we managed to fetch San Carlos without the need to tack in the heavy winds and seas. We eased our way into the bay and were shocked to find ourselves in only 11 feet of water while still a half-mile away from shore. With difficulty we tried following the coordinates to an anchorage given to us by a friend. Lack of sleep and confusion over where to anchor caused us to fumble through our usual procedures for dropping the main and the halyard wrapped around the steaming light, midway up the mast. Hungry and tired, we decided to tackle it in the morning. We spent a rocky night with 20-plus knot winds still blowing, no protection and still no fish for Norm. The next day, Norm went up the mast in the bosun's chair, retrieving the halyard so we could set forth again.

Later in the day, the wind and seas began to lie down, this time for good. We were out of the maelstrom, which most refer to as the "Baja Bash." As we approached Bahia San Quintin, Norm began to anticipate flagging down a *panga* to barter for a ride to shore and to swap our cans of chicken for fresh fish. Miles in advance of our arrival we optimistically began practicing our Spanish to secure a

126

round-trip (*ida y vuelta*) ride into town, as well as a sampling of the *panguera*'s catch. We planned in great detail how many and what type of fish we'd like to buy, how to prepare it, etc. When we arrived, we found ours to be the only boat in sight.

The next evening we anchored near Punta Colnett on our final overnight. It looked as though Norm would never get a bite of fresh fish. Again, there was a dearth of passing fishermen. Where was the much-anticipated parade of *pangas*? In desperation I hauled out the fishing gear. It was a wasted effort. No fish wandered over the sandy bottom.

Just as we were giving up hope, we spotted one lonely skiff carrying three, yellow mack-clad *hombres* approaching from the outer waters. We did everything short of sending up a flare to hail them and they approached at last. The eldest of them held their tossing boat off from our rail, its peeling turquoise paint threatening our spotless white fiberglass in the chop. We quickly dropped a bucket over the side into which they deposited a beautiful fish, which we believed to be an ocean whitefish. Immediately, they pushed off, refusing payment of any kind. Norm gestured to them wildly. There we were on the deck, waving cans of chicken in a vain effort to entreat them to return. They considerately paddled away from our boat, before starting their motor.

We were humbled. They'd had a long day, working in the cold in a small, pitching boat. Yet, they'd altered their course home for us, giving us part of their livelihood as a gift and left with broad smiles. "*Vaya con Dios*," Sharon yelled as their outboard kicked into gear. She was rewarded with broad grins – gracious and lovely smiles you could probably have seen all the way to San Diego.

On our last leg, as we motored through calm waters traveling the 63 miles from Punta Colnett to the Hotel Coral Marina, Norm suggested we 'debrief' to see what we'd learned during these 10 days. I took the task very seriously and began working on a lengthy list, shaming the rest of the crew into organizing their thoughts on paper. We were glad we did. It was a worthwhile exercise. Our discoveries included what we'd learned about our communications systems, such as using the marine single sideband radio and receiving GRIB files from NOAA on Sailmail, a myriad of computer

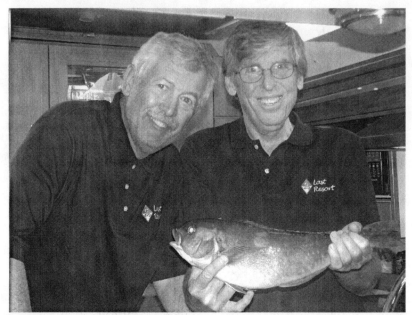

Norm's Turtle Bay "dream" comes true!

items shared between Norm and me, some housekeeping tips Charlene and Sharon swapped and lots of other practical items, in general. One great lesson Sharon and I learned is that we can be confident in the seaworthiness of our new boat.

Norm and Charlene proved themselves ready for anything, despite battling 30-knot winds, chilly temperatures, seasickness and threatening conditions. We mused after the trip that we hope they derived the same sense of accomplishment and satisfaction that we did. At the very least, we can report with absolute assuredness: Norm relished the great fish bestowed on us by the fishermen of Punta Colnett.

We had completed our first major passage aboard *Last Resort*. Soon we would be returning to the United States and making final preparations for the transition from part-time sailors to full-time cruisers.

Chapter 5
Repatriation

While we thoroughly enjoyed our time in Mexico, we were ready to return home to Southern California. We missed our old friends, we wanted to join in our yacht club cruises, and more than anything, we wanted to finish the work on the boat so we could close up our house in Scottsdale and finally move aboard.

In late June 2007, we drove from Arizona to Los Angeles on our last trip. We left our car at the Catalina dealership in Marina del Rey, California and joined some friends who were driving down to spend the weekend on their boat, which was also kept at the Coral Hotel Marina. For the next few days we made a point of entertaining all of our friends before we said our fond and sometimes tearful goodbyes. I'll never forget what one of the dock boys said to me as we left, "Thank you for your tips and your friendly." I knew it wouldn't be too long before we'd be returning.

Finally, on June 30, we left with our spirits high at the prospect of finally sailing in our beloved home waters, where it all began for me almost 50-years earlier. Seven months to the day since we first arrived, we sailed out of the Coral Hotel Marina. In one of those amazing coincidences that happen every now and then, less than an hour out, we got a radio call from a boat telling us to look behind us. I couldn't believe it, but there were our dear friends, John and Nancy, in their 54-foot powerboat, *La Sirena*, not more than a quarter-mile off our stern quarter. Imagine John traveling all the way from Cabo San Lucas and catching up with us just as we departed the Coral Hotel Marina.

We were heading for the Coronado Islands. I had only visited those islands once before, during the short time I had *Venus Butterfly* in San Diego. It's not legal to simply anchor there and sail back to the United States, because as soon as you drop an anchor, you've technically entered Mexico. In those days, I was pretty terrified of the Mexican rules and regulations, so we had just sailed out to the islands, cruised around a little bit and left immediately. But during the delivery from Marina del Rey to Ensenada, Captain Mark told us he frequently stops there overnight and that it is a good anchorage. I was eager to see the islands again and sample the anchorage for myself.

The weather was beautiful, so I knew the overnight stay would be calm. As we approached the anchorage, we had the opportunity to observe the aqua-farm operations. What were once proud fishing vessels had been transformed into bait barges and mother ships to the *pangas* that deliver the bait food to the large pens where tuna and other fish are grown.

Upon our arrival, we anchored well away from a boat that was already occupying the anchorage. A few minutes later, for no apparent reason, the skipper weighed anchor and moved to a spot dead in front of us. He did have the courtesy to inquire if I thought he was too close, probably because it was obvious. When I responded that I would sleep better if he moved, he pulled up anchor and moved a little farther away. During the afternoon, several more vessels anchored, but all were well clear. The anchorage was very calm and we slept well.

Getting a reasonably early start the next day, we saw quite a few dolphins on the short 20-mile trip to the U.S. Customs dock on Shelter Island. I never tire of cavorting dolphins and seeing them always reminds me of a favorite quote of mine from *The Hitchhikers Guide to the Galaxy*, "...on the planet Earth, man had always assumed that he was more intelligent than dolphins because he had achieved so much - the wheel, New York, wars and so on - while all the dolphins had ever done was muck about in the water having a good time. But conversely, the dolphins had always believed that they were far more intelligent than man - for precisely the same reasons."

Our plan was to leave the Coronado Islands in the morning so that we could clear U. S. Customs before the afternoon rush. We arrived at the Customs dock around 11:00 a.m. and cleared quickly. We'd learned that having and completing the form in advance can expedite the process. As soon as we were cleared, we proceeded the short distance to the Southwestern Yacht Club.

We maintain two yacht club memberships in order to maximize our reciprocity at participating yacht clubs. We had timed our arrival to coincide with the fleet from the Marina del Rey to San Diego Race. A number of friends from the Santa Monica Windjammers Yacht Club were participating and we were excited to greet them as they arrived. After almost all the other boats had arrived, we went up to the clubhouse to await the arrival of our friends, Joe and Sharon aboard their boat *Lucky Lady Too*, who finally dragged in at about 9:00 p.m. They were pretty wiped out, but we managed to tease them just a little about their "scientific" racing technique. Joe's buddy who had gone along as tactician had tried out a theory that burning incense and watching how the smoke flowed would help him read the wind. One had to conjecture since they were almost dead last to arrive, that it did not.

The next day, we entered Oceanside Harbor, unaware of the misfortune that would soon befall us. When I first tried to pull up to the check-in dock, both the current and wind were very strong and I had to make a second approach. I was still getting used to docking the boat in very different situations. In Mexico, the only dock I ever used was in our marina, since everywhere else required anchoring. So while our anchoring skills were excellent, I still needed a lot more practice docking. Oceanside assigned us to a very difficult dock located directly in front of the Jolly Roger Restaurant. On our first landing attempt we were blown off this dock as well, partly because I didn't have enough room to set up a proper approach. In hindsight, I should have backed in. I have since learned that with a bow thruster, it is far easier to back into tight quarters since the stern is far more responsive and the bow thruster takes care of the forward end of the boat.

We ended up having a really lovely visit with some friends from Scottsdale who maintain a beach front condominium right in the Oceanside Marina. One highlight of the visit was a ride in the Boston Whaler out into the big swells that were forming across the entrance bar. This would be my last joyride in the Whaler, since we had also made up our minds to sell it. We left with a promise to make plans to get them up to Marina del Rey for a sail on *Last Resort*.

The next morning, disaster struck. As we were pulling out of the dock, I simply ran out of maneuvering room and at the same moment the bow thruster failed. So I had to back right up to the breakwater. As it turned out, I got too close and the rudder smashed against the rocky bottom. When I started forward again the current drove us into the end of the dock where the steel frame surrounding a piling slit an ugly, deep gash in the port side of the boat. I was heartsick about this and definitely did not want to show up for the yacht club's return cruise at the Isthmus with this damage.

We ran into difficulties finding a place to moor after we finally got out of the ill-fated Oceanside Harbor. Newport Harbor, our next logical stop, was totally overbooked for the Fourth of July holiday, which I hadn't really considered when timing our departure from Mexico. Having no luck securing a guest mooring anywhere, and having made repeated phone calls, we ultimately decided to anchor in the public anchorage. After experimenting, we finally deployed two Danforth-type anchors, because our standard anchor wouldn't hold in the soft mud bottom. We enjoyed a very balmy and peaceful night. Unfamiliar with the anchorage, we didn't expect the rank-smelling, sludgy mud that covered our anchors and got all over the foredeck and cockpit when we retrieved them the next morning. It took almost an hour to clean up the mess with our internal wash-down system.

While we were still in Newport, we had spoken with Gary and learned that he had found us an end-tie moorage in Alamitos Bay. Shortly after our arrival, he and his fiancée Barbara, showed up to take possession of their 'new' dinghy. We were both very sad to watch as they left in our trusted Boston Whaler.

During his visit, Gary made arrangements for us to get the Gel-coat damage repaired. But later, turning the boat around to get the damaged side next the dock became another ordeal. Sharon was to stay on the dock and secure a stern line to a cleat so I could simply pivot the boat with the bow thruster. That might have worked if the bow thruster hadn't decided to die halfway through the maneuver. Sharon almost injured herself when she had a grip of the stern line just inches from the cleat and couldn't hold the boat anymore in the strong wind. Seeing this, I forgot everything else and backed down to try to relieve the pressure on the line. That worked and I decided to just motor out to make a new approach. The near-injury had scared us both, bringing Sharon to tears for a little while.

The next morning, the fiberglass repair team showed up. By 12:30 p.m. they had completed such a magnificent repair you would have never known the accident happened. Only Gary, Sharon and the repair guys knew that it had happened at all and we weren't going to tell.

With the repair completed and the Boston Whaler gone, we headed over to the Isthmus at Catalina to hook up with the returning Marina del Rey to San Diego Race fleet. The wind was already blowing 15 knots and without the Boston Whaler dragging behind us, we were really making good time and completed the trip in well under four hours. The same trip in our old Catalina 36 used to take almost six hours and we were really starting to appreciate the speed of the new boat.

This was a star-graced trip that would have a profound effect on me and shape my life for a long time to come. Sharon wrote about it in an article entitled "Meeting the Grand Poobah." Here are some excerpts about meeting Richard, publisher of *Latitude 38* – San Francisco's go-to sailor's rag – and self-styled Grand Poobah of the annual fun-rally down the west coast of Mexico, the Baja Ha-Ha:

> Twenty years, several shirt-sizes (and one wife) earlier, my husband, Captain Dick, had submitted an article to San Francisco's legendary sailing magazine, *Latitude 38*, and was given a "Roving Reporter" tee-shirt. "Do we have the Roving Reporter shirt?" he's now asking me.
>
> "What's the emergency?" I ask as I rummage through my locker. Of course I have it. It's my favorite tee-shirt, well-worn, roomy and a great color. (Of course, you have to overlook the bleach splotch around the navel area where I unfortunately leaned into my cleaning.) It's my lucky hand-me-down, now that it no longer fits Dick.
>
> "Richard, the publisher, is here at the Isthmus! Put it on and come along so we can show him. It's an antique and I think he'll get a kick out of it!"
>
> When we spot activity aboard Richard's catamaran, *Profligate,* we blast our way over, hardly able to restrain

ourselves from speeding through the no-wake zone. "Ahoy, there!" Dick shouts, waving our shirt like a burgee. And there he is…Richard.

Richard welcomes us aboard for an impromptu sail. He doesn't know a stranger. "You want to come out for a sail?" he asks. My gosh! We feel we've been invited aboard a magic carpet ride. Richard may be at the helm, but it turns out the real captain is his significant other, Doña, an exotic beauty wrapped in a sarong and handing out assignments to the crew. A commercially licensed sea captain (up to 100 tons), she divides her time between orchestrating the preparations for her own birthday celebration and managing the sail. Richard encourages me during my turn at the wheel as I reach for that afternoon's record of 12.6 knots (only held for a few more minutes as it turns out). I'll have bragging rights at the bar I am told. I am elated until I hear that means I'll be buying the first round! I'm pretty relieved when I am bested.

As we are wafted along on *Profligate's* enormous twin hulls, I have a moment to talk to Richard about the famous 750-mile rally-*cum*-race he shepherds each year from San Diego to Cabo San Lucas. I must confess at this point that I had arrived aboard Richard's boat more than a little awed by his reputation. People tend to speak of him as almost a mythical creature – a long-time bastion of the San Francisco sailing community and surpassing seaman: The Grand Poobah, who possesses all the mystique of *Der Fleigland Hollander* (whose fabled ghostly ship would rip past other vessels as they lay becalmed). But in Richard we find no Wagnerian dignitary, stooping to elevate with a bejeweled hand. He's just a guy – a fellow cruiser.

Our spirits are lifted by the conviviality of the hour and that evening we muse about the draw of our calling. We have experienced another example that it's more than the wheel's kick and the wind's song that lend the cruising life its allure; it has as much to do with the camaraderie of our fellow adventurers. The grandness of the Grand Poobah is that he, like us, is on this same journey, blown by the same winds, fair or otherwise. And in our own way, aren't we all Grand Poobahs of our vessels and destinies?

The rest of the trip wasn't quite as eventful, but we enjoyed it just the same, especially the USC Wrigley Science Foundation tour and the lecture about viruses and bacteria. We were interested to learn that 90 percent of the oxygen on earth is actually produced in the sea by these microscopic organisms. We had a nice dinner with our yacht club buddies, but they all seemed to be pretty worn out from the races. They were an unusually subdued lot that weekend.

Bob had arranged a slip for us in Marina del Rey, so we got an early start on July 8, 2007 and headed out around 9:00 a.m. The slip turned out to be a nightmare to get in and out of because our finger had a piling along side the outer edge which presented a real hazard when entering and leaving the slip. It wasn't a pretty landing and we managed to mar the hull. That's the cost of having a new boat; every scratch kills you. And of course, all of the nicks and bumps come when it's new and you're still learning the ropes.

Sharon had planned a trip to visit her daughter in Germany before we realized the Catalina Rendezvous, an annual gathering of owners sponsored by Catalina Yachts at Two Harbors, was to be held that very weekend. I was really counting on going to show off our new boat, so we invited some old friends, Sandra and Rick, to fly in from Virginia.

About an hour out of the harbor, as we pulled abeam of Palos Verdes Point, a large powerboat that had been passing about a quarter-mile to port suddenly changed course and was headed directly for us. This made Rick and Sandra pretty nervous. They were on watch as I was below decks trying to down my liquid lunch at precisely that moment. Once I determined that they were going to take my stern, I resumed lunch, only to be called topside a few moments later when Rick said we were being hailed. Well, lo and behold, it was the boat that was carrying Sharon, one of the senior executives at Catalina Yachts, to the Rendezvous. They circled us for some time to take pictures of *Last Resort*.

On the way over we saw a number of dolphins and seals, which Rick and Sandra seemed to thoroughly enjoy. Then, about half-way

135

through the trip, we were thrilled when we intercepted the TransPac Race fleet as they departed Point Fermin to make their way around the West End of Catalina Island, their only obstacle *en route* to Diamond Head in Honolulu, Hawaii. The TransPac race, first held in 1906, was inspired by King Kalakaua, the revered Hawaiian leader of the late 19th century who believed that such an event would strengthen the islands' economic and cultural ties to the mainland. By monitoring the VHF radio, we learned that the large, fast sled boats, as they are called, would be starting the same day we were leaving. We promptly decided to adjust our departure to intercept them as they were sailing between Long Beach and Catalina Island and get a glimpse of these ultra-fast giants.

As if we weren't already having an exceptional trip, with only five miles to go to Catalina, the wind kicked up to 20 knots and our speed increased to 8.6 knots, our theoretical hull speed. Hull speed is a mathematically derived number representing the maximum speed, outside factors such as following seas excluded, that a boat should be able to travel through the water. Sandra came back from a quick excursion below decks and said it was "…like *The Poseidon Adventure* down there!" Upon arrival, the crew did a masterful job of tying up to a mooring buoy in Cherry Cove. This is the most coveted mooring location on the entire island, but it turned out not to be as calm as advertised. We found it much more comfortable after we deployed the flopper stopper.

Of all things, it turned out Rick played the bagpipe. To my bemusement, he said that "If I play, they will come." I didn't believe him until during his impromptu concert from the foredeck, as he played a number of traditional bagpipe tunes, the haunting tones of his solo concert drew eager listeners from every direction.

Once he'd proved what a draw the bagpipe was, Rick and I cooked up a plan. Later that evening, Rick led Sandra and me into the cocktail party to a military cadence on his pipe as we fell in behind. This had to be the grandest of all entrances I have ever made. I had clued Charlene to tell Norm to have his camera ready, so fortunately he made a short clip of our arrival, which I subsequently posted on YouTube. It was truly a sight to behold and people were talking about it for a long time following the event.

136

Rick and Sandra left the party on the early side, but I was glad I didn't leave with them, because in the raffle I won a second folding lounge seat for our cockpit. Riding alone in the dinghy all the way to Cherry Cove in two-foot swells and lots of headwind on a pitch black night was a little scary, especially being Friday the 13th.

The next day, Rick had promised some of our neighbors there would be another bagpipe concert that afternoon at 4:30 p.m. Again there was a crowd; coming by dinghy and kayak, watching from the decks of their nearby boats and even one guy who actually swam over to personally request *Amazing Grace*.

There were over 200 people at the Rendezvous, but I had a chance to visit with Frank, the owner of Catalina Yachts. He was most interested and sympathetic to my health issues and swallowing disorder and we managed to bond during that short visit. Rick, Sandra and I relived more of the glory of the bagpipe entrance from the night before, as person after person commented to us about it. Riding back on the shore boat I discovered just how helpful the solar cockpit lights were in finding our boat amongst hundreds of others in the crowded moorage. I had originally purchased marine-rated solar cockpit lights, but they only lasted about a month before failing during the heavy weather leaving Turtle Bay. The replacements from Home Depot were half the price and were holding up far better.

We had to return on Sunday so Rick and Sandra could catch their redeye flight to Virginia Beach at 10:30 p.m. This allowed us to delay our departure and intersect the maxi-sleds participating in the TransPac. The grand finale of the entire Catalina Rendezvous weekend came when we successfully met the TransPac fleet. The undeniable leader was Roy Disney's *Pyewacket*, a rocket-ship of a boat that had just undergone $2 million in modifications to increase its original 86-foot length to more than 90 feet in preparation for the TransPac Race.

I was sorry to see Rick and Sandra depart for the airport, but was looking forward to Sharon's return. The next few months would be the busiest we'd had in many a year. On Monday, I met with Bob and Byron and scheduled an aggressive plan to finally finish off the boat. Based on our experience, which now spanned well over a year and hundreds of sailing miles, we had made the final equipment and modification decisions. Over the next two months the boat's interior would be torn apart one more time, hopefully the last, to accommodate the work.

In July, I also received an irresistible invitation from Richard, publisher of *Latitude 38*, whom we'd met a month before and with whom we were becoming friends. He emailed to ask if I'd like to crew for him in the Santa Barbara to King Harbor Race. I hadn't crewed in a race in many years, so I jumped at the opportunity. The weekend of the race, Sharon drove me to Santa Barbara where we stayed in a cozy little bed and breakfast near the harbor. That night we joined Richard and the other participants at the pre-race cocktail party hosted by the Santa Barbara Yacht Club.

The race was sailed in mostly light air and I was assigned the job of trimming the spinnaker. I hadn't flown a spinnaker since my racing days on Lake Tahoe and the thrill of having that tiger by the tail again convinced me that we should order a cruising spinnaker for *Last Resort*. The winds died out completely during the night, so at around 1:00 a.m. Richard decided to retire from the race and motor into King Harbor, since by that point our GPS track showed us dead in the water.

During the course of the race, I had the opportunity to talk one-on-one with each of Richard's friends, including Shannon, a very personable and attractive young woman who took an immediate interest in my story. I wasn't big on telling people about my affliction, but it was apparent to everyone aboard that I wasn't eating or drinking. When pressed, I told Shannon the whole story. I wasn't aware of it at the time, but she had been so moved that she relayed my whole story to Richard the following day.

A couple of weeks after the Santa Barbara to King Harbor Race, I received a call from Doña, Richard's significant other and partner of 11 years. She said that Richard wanted to do a story about me and wondered if I could provide the magazine with a recent photograph. I didn't have one readily available, but since we were moored at Catalina, there were lots of scenic places to take a picture, so I told her I'd get her something before the day was out. I posed for a shot of myself at the helm and promptly sent it off by email.

A few days later, Richard himself called to say that he had some questions he'd like to ask. Would I mind spending a few minutes on the phone with him? He relayed to me that Shannon had told him my story, which he was writing in an article for the magazine, and needed to fill in some blanks. After hearing the entire story over the course of the next half-hour, Richard said he'd decided to write a more comprehensive article to give the story more prominence in the magazine. As the date of publication for the August issue drew near I was becoming more and more interested in seeing just what he might have written. I started going to the West Marine store in Marina del Rey every day starting August 1. On August 4 the issue finally arrived and I was honored that my story had received prominent placement. After the story appeared, I received dozens of calls and emails. One email was particularly moving,

> "Thank you, for your awesome story in *Latitude 38* this month, it has inspired me even further to continue my current track. The reason this story means so much to me is that I had my last chemo treatment for throat cancer approximately seven weeks ago. My wife and I have been living on our 47-foot wooden ketch. We have been actively engaged in getting ready to cruise extensively, but the cancer was a severe setback, making me question all of my decisions. My throat has healed very well to this point and I am eating by mouth most foods that can be macerated or blended to a consistency of mashed potatoes. I can almost swallow a pea without choking. It does continue to improve but I still have a feeding tube. Your commitment to sailing/cruising has inspired me to continue with my life long dream. Thank you, Dan"

Richard made mention in the article that I had a website and included the URL in the story. Back when we had first made the decision to buy the boat and ultimately take off cruising, I had wanted to start a website to keep my immediate family and close friends apprised of our travels. I had never designed or created a website before, but I was anxious to learn. It was a hole in my resume that I thought I should fill anyway, so I set about learning the process. It turned out that Verio, who hosted my business websites, had an easy template-based program that was fairly straightforward to use. So in my usual compulsive manner, I set aside 24 straight hours to design, write and edit a website. Much to my incredulity, in half that time, I actually had my own website, www.voyagesoflastresort.com, up and running.

I was so excited I broadened my mailing list, and before long, had approximately 150 people I would email as changes and updates were posted. Sharon and I had been very busy and it was never a problem to find content for the website, which I usually updated with a major redo of the home page every two months or so. One day while I was tinkering with the software I discovered a hit counter. When I looked at it the first time, I couldn't believe my eyes. There had been slightly over 12,000 hits in the first three months. How could this be, I wondered? In an effort to determine where all these hits were coming from, I happened to bring the subject up to one of my oncologists in Scottsdale. He said that he was telling all his patients about my website, as well as my doctors in Texas. In the beginning, I made no mention of my affliction with cancer or the difficult treatment and recovery that I had experienced on my site. It had been strictly devoted to sailing and stories of our adventures aboard *Last Resort*. But, apparently Larry and his seriously ill neighbor were not the only ones who found my story inspiring. The Internet is an amazing resource and word of my story was spreading virally.

Much to my amazement, the month the story appeared in *Latitude 38*, I received over 50,000 hits. I was beginning to realize that my story might actually be resonating, providing hope and inspiration to a large number of people. I started to wonder how I might be able to do something even more significant, and over the next few months, Sharon and I would have this discussion on a recurring basis.

In the meantime, we had made the final decision to install the watermaker aboard *Last Resort*. Having had the experience of running out of water in Turtle Bay, we realized that we must have a watermaker to do any serious international cruising. The hottest-selling model at the time, according to the Catalina dealer, was the Spectra Newport II. This unit had the advantage of a self-timing flush mechanism that would allow the unit to go unused for long periods of time without the need for it to be totally disabled and pickled. We decided to install it right away and worked out a schedule with the Newport Beach-based supplier.

That decision led us to another one. With a watermaker aboard, we could eliminate one of the five water tanks that were standard on the boat. We didn't like carrying extra fuel on deck or dealing with jerry jugs on the Turtle Bay trip, so another lesson learned was that we needed more inboard fuel capacity. We'd decided to replace the inoperative 62-gallon water storage tank with a factory-optional fuel tank, which would boost our fuel capacity to approximately 135 gallons and ensure an operational range, under motor power alone, well in excess of 500 miles. We would be free of the cumbersome jerry jugs, which I later sold.

We needed to haul *Last Resort* to have the rudder repaired, because our diver had reported some damage that occurred when we hit the rocks along the seawall in Oceanside. We decided it would also be a good time to install a folding propeller. I'd never had one before, but all the other Catalina 470s participating on the Association's message board that had them raved about their performance. After doing a lot of research, I decided on a Gori folding, two-blade propeller. This unit had the advantage of offering two speeds of operation, standard and overdrive. In overdrive we found we could easily maintain 7.2 knots with the engine running at only 2400 rpm, resulting in almost a thirty percent drop in fuel consumption.

The fuel tank and watermaker installations took almost a month to complete. During that month, while the boat was torn apart and the work was being supervised by Byron, whom we trusted implicitly to carry on the job in our absence, we traveled to Scottsdale.

We had made the pivotal decision to take the final leap. While my health was still questionable, my recent scans had all been clear and I hadn't needed to have my throat dilated in over six months.

We loved living aboard the boat and knew it was time to start the arduous process of closing up the house. It had already been on the market for over a year, but an economic downturn was beginning and there were no buyers around. We were toying with the idea of keeping the house as an investment and renting it until the market could rebound and we could realize a profit. The difficulty was that the income which would be generated by the invested proceeds from the sale of the house was an important part of our retirement strategy. Renting out the house was a partial answer. As the economic conditions, particularly in the housing market, were worsening to near-record proportions, the reality was that Sharon would need to continue working and I would have to find other means to supplement our income, perhaps for several years to come.

Between us, we had combined two households and belongings that were accumulated over a number of years. All that stuff seemed important to us before, but we were sure we could easily live without almost all of it once we moved aboard ship. It wasn't a sudden realization, however, and we had to ease our way there. We started out with a garage sale and only put things which we really didn't want on display. We were surprised to learn that one man's junk is apparently another man's treasure and things were being snatched up in frenzy. We soon started hauling out more stuff and adding to our financial coffers. At the end of the day, we had several thousand dollars to show for our efforts, and a whole lot less 'stuff,' which we soon found we didn't even really need.

When we went back into the house to collect our thoughts and review our progress from that first sale, we realized that we still hadn't even scratched the surface. So next came a long period while we made pass after pass through the house, garbage bags at the ready, to toss out stuff we thought had no value and we could live without. Reassessing our situation, we decided we would need another garage sale. We still had too many things we knew we couldn't keep, but which were just too good to end up in the trash pile.

In the meantime, the work on the boat was progressing and it was time to return to Marina del Rey to prepare the boat for the haul-out. A few days later it was time to take the boat to the yard. Our adventure started early – at 7:30 a.m. – as we dodged UCLA rowing teams to get to the Windward Boat Yard and 'beat the crowd.' We were told it's first-come, first-served. We were first, all right. We were also last, since no other boats came during the entire day. Finally, around noon, we were besieged by five fast-moving dock hands who promptly shooed us off the boat and immediately started pulling her by her dock lines into position under the travel lift. We joked that the Windward crew was as organized as a suntan lotion vendor in a nudist resort. When we saw the huge hoist, it seemed unmanned, ghosting across the yard. It was actually being guided by a guy who wielded a remote control like a teenager with a Nintendo game. I'd never seen this boat hoisted before and fascinated, I videotaped the whole scene.

No sooner had they lowered *Last Resort* onto her keel, than they propped her up on what looked to be a few strategically-positioned toothpicks. Finally, there she sat, with her deck 13 feet above the very solid and unforgiving-looking concrete. We were a little timid as we picked our way up the ladder for the first time to enter our suspended home. That night we had a rough time sleeping. Sharon said she felt like we were living in a big box balanced over what could very well be ground zero of 'the big one.' This was, after all, earthquake country. We needn't have worried, as the supports were assembled with care and solidly in place. It was a good thing, because Marina del Rey was in for some unusually violent fall weather.

Ever since I was a young child, I have always feared lightning. I've heard many stories over the years of the devastating results of lightning strikes, especially on boats, including one fellow sailor who was hit by lightning at Lake Tahoe and never fully recovered. Sharon still laughs when she tells the story of attending a party, four houses down from our Scottsdale home, during a monsoon-season storm. There was so much lightning that I was afraid to walk the 400 feet to the neighbor's house, so I actually drove us there, convinced it was too dangerous to leave ourselves exposed to the searing bolts of lightning overhead. Sharon, who had a lot more experience with lightning, thought I was crazy and told me

143

so. I'll admit, I felt a little silly backing the car home at the end of that evening.

This would be our first experience living on the hard, and in addition to the logistical problems this presented, we soon found ourselves in the middle of an unusual series of fall thunderstorms that brought gale force winds and actual lightning – all but unheard of for Marina del Rey. Our mast normally rises 65 feet from the waterline, but on shore, our deep keel added an additional eight feet to the height, so we were like the Sears Tower, dominating everything else in the neighborhood. We spent one hair-raising night aboard as the boat vibrated under the reverberating rig while it was battered by the fierce winds threatening to topple us over at any moment. The lightning bolts looked like they were taking aim at our mast-*cum*-lightning-rod, closing in from every direction. We were most relieved when the storm passed, but only after we spent a tense five hours in fear of the danger broiling all around us. So passed our second night on the hard.

The next day the work began in earnest. There was Gelcoat work to be done in the cockpit, the rudder needed work and our shiny, new Gori prop, looking more like a piece of finely sculptured bronze than a rugged, heavy duty piece of marine equipment, needed to be fitted and installed on the shaft. We were putting pressure on Catalina Yachts to have the local representative of the bow thruster manufacturer come by the boatyard to inspect the unit and determine why it was consistently shutting off at critical moments during difficult docking procedures, such as the failure that led to the accident in Oceanside.

I have always believed that it's foolish to have work done in a boatyard if you can't be present. One day, however, while we were still in the yard, we were diverted by a business matter. The Gelcoat work in the cockpit had required removing the engine instrument panel. I had one of my better laughs when I returned that evening to find it re-installed, only upside down. I got such a kick out of it I forwarded a picture to *Latitude 38*, which ran it a month later in the online '*Lectronic Latitude*.'

Living on the hard for a week presented other problems. You couldn't really use the shower or the sinks, as the gray water would

144

drain directly onto the ground, so we used the guest bathroom in the yard, where Sharon had to cart all her dishes to wash them as well. Fortunately the facilities were first rate and very well-maintained, so showering in the yard was not a serious inconvenience. The boat's heads pumped into holding tanks, so they were no problem, and just like our dock, the marina had shore power hook ups, providing enough power for all our electronics, television, and the rest.

The bow thruster representative finally agreed to make the trip from his Newport Beach office to Marina del Rey. He arrived early in the morning and after inspecting the unit, suggested that the brushes were worn and said he would take it up with the manufacturer. I was by now on very good terms with Frank, the owner of Catalina Yachts, and while I hated to use up a favor, this issue warranted some intervention. I believed the problem with the unit was far more serious and after I described all the difficulties we'd had to Frank, he agreed to personally call to get a better resolution of the issue. That's all it took, because within a half-hour, I received a call that before the day was out we would have a replacement bow thruster installed. You can probably start figuring out about now why I've had a 25-year love affair with Catalina Yachts.

The work took what seemed like one, very long, week to complete, but finally the day came when *Last Resort* would be "splashed," a term the yard likes to use for launching a boat. After she was gently returned to her natural habitat, we motored back across the channel to our new slip. Finding a slip in Marina del Rey had been a long search. A new 227-slip marina and apartment complex was being constructed at the time and required closing the old marina and dislodging all the tenants. Acute demand was placed on an already over-taxed supply of available slips, especially since the original opening date was already six months behind schedule. I appealed to the dockmaster at the California Yacht Club with whom I'd become friends, and through his efforts, found a sublease opportunity. One of my fellow club members was in the practice of spending the winter in Mexico, so his slip became available from August through March. The timing couldn't have been better. It was a 60-foot slip and pretty pricy, but it also fronted on the main channel and afforded us an entertaining perch from which to watch the goings-on in the harbor.

During the months of September, October and November, we divided our time equally between Scottsdale and sailing in Southern California. During this time we had the opportunity to entertain a large number of my old friends and take many of them sailing. We had also narrowed the house-clearing process down to nothing more than the big pieces of furniture and personal belongings, family heirlooms and artwork that we intended to keep. The cheapest storage we could find was in Palm Springs and we managed to pare down our remaining belongings to fit into a 10-by-10-foot air-conditioned storage locker.

The logistics can seem overwhelming when you decide to permanently cut the dock lines and transition to a full-time life of living and cruising aboard ship. Mail handling and forwarding was a concern, so we rented a mail box from the local Scottsdale UPS Store. This gave us the dual advantages of being able to maintain a normal street address in Arizona and having our mail forwarded periodically to whatever port in which we might find ourselves.

We were determined to maximize our time in Southern California and visit all of the various ports where we had friends to bid farewell, knowing we'd be gone for a very long time, once we finally left. Ever since we'd become aware that climate change was reportedly accelerating the melting of the glaciers, we'd settled on Alaska as our first destination. We also wanted to get as much of our cold-weather sailing behind us as possible before we got too much older.

Included on our must-see list was a cruise to the Channel Islands off the coast of Santa Barbara. We had stopped there once a few years before, but that short stop only whetted our appetite for a lengthier exploration. I'd also been by there while crewing in the Santa Barbara to King Harbor race, which rounded Anacapa Island as part of the race course, and I was again lured by the intrigue of these islands.

So one Friday in October, we carved out two weeks to cruise and explore these islands. Just prior to our departure, the Coast Guard issued a warning for gale force Santa Ana winds and seas to 15 feet in the Santa Barbara Channel for that night, extending through Monday and maybe even Tuesday.

We were delayed in our departure due to the discovery that the luff tape which fits inside the mast track was separating from the mainsail at the second batten from the top, creating the risk of a complete failure if not repaired immediately. Sharon did a great job stitching an emergency repair so we could get underway. We decided to detour to Channel Islands Harbor where I'd made arrangements for Ullman Sails to replace the luff tape, which had been completely redesigned and would be changed at no cost to us.

Given the weather report and our delayed departure, we decided we would only sail as far as Paradise Cove, where we thought we'd get some protection if the seas built as forecast, yet remain close enough to Marina del Rey to easily return if the winds did build to gale force.

Sharon's repair held-up well and we had no further problems with the sail, even with apparent winds close to 18 knots. *En route* to Paradise Cove we enjoyed steady winds, but as it got closer to sunset, they subsided and we motor-sailed the last three miles. It took two tries to get the anchor set. I believed we were anchored too far out the first time to be fully protected, so the second attempt was far more successful and the anchor seemed to be holding, important if the forecast winds blew overnight.

You never know about the accuracy of Southern California weather forecasts, because more times than not, rain or other forecast conditions just don't seem to materialize. This night the forecasters would prove to be accurate. When the wind was blowing a steady 45 knots, with one 53-knot gust recorded by our anemometer, the anchor finally refused to maintain its tenuous hold on the seaweed-laden bottom. We had no choice but to haul it up and make a run back to Marina del Rey. We finally got the anchor off the bottom after 45 minutes of effort, only to discover it was wrapped up in hundreds of pounds of seaweed. Our efforts to raise it out of the water onto the bow roller repeatedly resulted in an overloaded circuit as the windlass strained beyond its 400-pound limit. We were quickly being blown offshore and our efforts to sail with this slimy mass anchored to the bow were futile. We

147

finally had to heave to (arrange the sails in such a manner as to slow or stop the forward motion of the boat, such as when in heavy seas) and clear off the seaweed. Working on the bow with the boat hook, I was pelted by sheets of sea spray blowing from atop the tumultuous waves as we slowly drifted farther offshore. After a solid hour, I finally cleared the last of the seaweed from the anchor. Once done, we were able to head back to Marina del Rey. Due to the strong gusting winds and heavy seas, we were only making about five knots. It was turning out to be a very long night.

By 4:00 a.m. we were moving along at about six knots, the best we'd been able to achieve. The farther offshore we sailed, the more the increasing fetch allowed the seas to build. The winds were still at a steady 30 knots and we were constantly jostled about. We were starting to experience occasional pounding as our hull was launched from the tops of the steep, six-foot waves.

This was my second experience navigating from primarily below decks, using the autopilot remote control from my calm, dry perch at the chart table. With the large radar display and other tools at my disposal at the navigation station, I could work in the comfort of the cabin, just sticking my head up every once in a while to check for other boat traffic or obstacles the radar might miss.

By about 5:00 a.m. the winds had picked up again and were gusting to 35 knots. I suspected we were getting a funnel effect from Malibu Canyon. We continued to be knocked about and our speed had dropped below five knots. As we passed Malibu Canyon we glimpsed an orange glow that lit up the hillsides in the predawn darkness. Clearly, a huge fire had started. We were out of cell phone range and unsure whom, if anyone, a 911-call on the satellite phone would reach. I therefore turned immediately to my hand-held ham radio. I was a member of a Southern California network of radio repeaters and tuned to their different frequencies until I heard a conversation in progress, which I immediately interrupted with my emergency traffic. I asked if they would please report the fire. They were aware of a network that maintained a 24/7 fire watch during Santa Ana wind conditions and agreed to make immediate contact. I monitored the conversations and it wasn't long until we spotted the flashing red lights of a convoy of fire trucks snaking along the Pacific Coast Highway. This fire quickly became a huge conflagration. Some weeks later we were surprised to learn from a friend that the media reported the original fire alarm had been raised by a sailboat using a ham radio off the Malibu shore. I knew from my radar watch and the adverse conditions, we were likely the only sailors foolhardy enough to have been out at that time in those seas.

We finally made it into our slip a little after 6:30 a.m. The seas and winds were almost dead calm when we arrived back at Marina del Rey, an amazing fact considering the conditions we had left only 10 miles behind. A morning-after inspection revealed lots of crystallized salt on the boat, but no damage. It had turned out to be a wise decision not to push on to the Channel Islands, where the seas quickly reached 20 feet, although perhaps a wiser decision would have been to not go at all until we knew if the winds were really going to materialize as forecast. Another lesson learned.

In the ensuing 72 hours since we limped back to Marina del Rey, Southern California experienced the worst fire storms in history, starting with this fire we'd spotted. At one point on Monday night, 15 fires were raging from Ventura to San Diego counties, over 1500 homes and businesses had been lost and an amazing 500,000 people had lost their homes or been evacuated from the paths of the fires. The Governor and the President had declared a State of Emergency in Southern California. Miraculously, only one person had reportedly died. Malibu, which we observed first hand on our way back to Marina del Rey Sunday morning, only lost six homes and a church. The Arrowhead area (including Green Valley Lake where our friend Byron has his home) as well as Orange County and San Diego, in particular, took the worst of it. My sister's house in San Diego County, as well as Byron's house, were both miraculously spared, but many of their friends and neighbors were not so lucky.

With the exception of this tragic incident, the six months we spent in Southern California aboard *Last Resort* were some of the best times I can remember. I was encouraged by the steady improvement in the condition of my throat. One nurse had suggested that the humidity of the marine environment could explain the dramatic improvement. The following January, I was scheduled for another battery of tests and scans. The doctors had been watching a small spot on one of my lungs. My particular brand of cancer, if it metastasized, would likely spread first to my lungs, so the nagging tug of dread was always with me as these months rolled by. Fortunately, we were so busy that I didn't have much time to dwell on those thoughts.

When we finally resumed our aborted Channel Islands cruise a week later, the conditions couldn't have been better. After a brief overnight stop in Channel Islands Harbor near Oxnard, followed by a stop at the Santa Barbara Yacht Club, we were finally off to explore the islands. Our first stop would be Cuyler Harbor on San Miguel Island, one of the farthest anchorages and the most exposed to the northerly winds and seas that prevail all summer. When we'd sailed far enough out to be clear of the lee of Point Conception, the wind picked up and we were able to set the jib, increasing our speed to a steady 8.5 knots.

We arrived and found the harbor to be much larger than we had envisioned. We anchored in 24 feet of water. An otherwise perfect anchoring job was marred by the fact that Sharon lost her voice activated radio overboard while she was struggling on the foredeck. We had enough practice by now that I was confident we could anchor using just hand signals, so we didn't worry too much about it. I was more distressed by the fact that the hands-free radio set had been a gift from our friends John and Nancy, but it turned out to be an easy thing to replace. The harbor itself had a beautiful, scenic shoreline with long sandy beaches punctuated by dramatic rock outcrops.

A couple of other boats, *Just the Two of Us* with Mike and Ann aboard and *Last Mango* with Mike and Gladys, pulled in later that afternoon. Once they were settled we invited them all over for cocktails in the evening. It turns out they were both from Washington and were headed to the South Pacific. We gleaned some very useful tips about the Pacific Northwest from them and reciprocated with information we hoped would be helpful when they began cruising in Mexico. Both of the guys on the other boats were ham radio operators as well, so we decided to try making contact with their

150

ham radio network in the Pacific Northwest. We had some good luck with the radio, not only talking to our friends' Pacific Northwest-based ham net, but also responding successfully to two stations that were CQ contesting, or looking for as many contacts in as short a time as possible. We also found the BBC news on 7160MHz, although we lost that signal after about an hour of catching up with world affairs.

The next morning, we made radio contact and were introduced to Barbara, who runs the Great Northern Boaters Net every morning, year-round at 8:00 a.m. This was an important contact because we would rely on the Great Northern Boaters Net to keep track of us once we reached the Pacific Northwest and ventured into even higher latitudes and the remote waters of northern British Columbia and Alaska. I also fine-tuned my communications techniques and successfully utilized Sailmail over the new Iridium satellite phone's data modem, thanks to the Ocens Internet service to which I'd subscribed.

When the winds picked up to 20 knots from the north the following morning, the anchorage became untenable, so we hurriedly departed. It was almost a straight downwind run to Santa Rosa Island, sailing wing-on-wing, jib and mainsail on opposite sides of the boat. When we rounded Carrington Point, we found ourselves on a beam reach doing 8.9 knots, a new sailing record, not counting the downwind sailing we'd done during our initial sea trial with Bob. On that trip we momentarily saw 12 knots as we surfed down the face of a large wave.

Bechers Bay was much calmer than Cuyler Harbor the first night we anchored there. It was prettier too. It sits off a broad expanse of white sand beach, much like Smuggler's Anchorage on Santa Cruz Island. The wind was blowing down the coast, rather than funneling through the canyons, so the heavy gusts were somewhat mitigated. It helped that the temperature reached 75° F. and the balmy winds felt almost tropical.

Enjoying the calm anchorage, we persuaded Mike and Gladys aboard *Last Mango* to come around and anchor near us, where we were sure they'd be more comfortable. Soon after their arrival, a large sea swell began to roll through the anchorage when the wind shifted, and it only got worse as the night went on. It was a very miserable night with large swells causing us to rock uncomfortably. We felt very sorry for Mike and Gladys in their smaller boat. When we awoke shortly after sunrise, we found they were already gone.

I had good success on the radio that morning and was able to make contact with Richard, who aboard his large catamaran *Profligate*, was shepherding the Baja Ha-Ha fleet as they made their way down the Baja coast, over 400 miles distant. We heard the roll call and relayed Don Anderson's weather report, which was broadcast from nearby Ventura, and which they had trouble receiving.

Due to the uncomfortable conditions in the anchorage, we too made a fast departure for the seven-mile passage across the Santa Cruz Channel. We tried an experiment sailing with just the jib, but soon found it didn't stabilize the boat at all in a beam sea. From then on, we always used the mainsail, unless we were doing a short run dead down wind in calm seas. At about 10:40 a.m. we put into Forney Cove. It was rough enough that we set the flopper stopper immediately upon arrival. Once that was deployed, the anchorage was quite pleasant. As I went to bed, I reported in the ship's log that it was a truly spectacular day. I'd made great strides in my ability to maximize communications with our high-tech satellite and radio gear, which would prove an invaluable asset during our subsequent cruising. I'd had a fruitful day on the ham radio, received some warm emails from friends, enjoyed a beautiful happy hour watching the sunset from the cockpit as the wind died down, and was able to capture some great photography. All in all, a pretty cool day!

The next day we awoke to a lovely sunny morning with only three knots of wind. I was up early so that I could again relay Don Anderson's weather report to Richard and the Baja Ha-Ha fleet. I raised Richard on the single sideband radio and passed along the weather, which he shared with the group during the roll call, graciously giving me credit. A little later I returned to single sideband radio, tuning back in just as one of the fleet reported receiving a digital distress call and capturing the ship's MMSI (Marine Mobile Service Identity) number, a digital signature that allows Coast Guard search and rescue personnel to identify the boat and its owner, but more importantly, their position, assuming they have taken the all-important step of connecting their radio to a GPS (Global Positioning System) receiver. I jumped into the conversation and for the next half-hour relayed information to the U.S. Coast Guard, both in San Diego and Los Angeles. Upon overhearing the communications, Gordon West, the West Coast ham radio guru with whose help and excellent classes we'd obtained our own ham licenses, chimed in to say that he would call them on a land line, presumably to offer his many years of emergency radio experience to assist in contacting the vessel in distress. MMSI numbers can be obtained directly from the FCC or through BoatUS. BoatUS's MMSI registration number service is free for boat owners that don't otherwise require FCC licensing. The Coast Guard maintains a central database of MMSI numbers, but training issues still occasionally result in confusion when Coast Guard personnel attempt to access the database in an emergency. We'd filed our station license application and received our MMSI number directly from the FCC when we received our ship's station license. I continued to monitor the communications over the next several days and ultimately the Coast Guard classified the report as a false alarm, because no boats were reported missing in the area and nothing further was heard.

During this trip, Sharon and I talked extensively about how I might be able to contribute to aid others afflicted with cancer. I came up with the idea to start a foundation similar to the Make-A-Wish Foundation, enlisting an armada of yachtsmen who would volunteer their boats to take a cancer patient and their friends or family out for a day sail to get some respite from the rigors of treatment in the aftermath of this insidious disease. From these discussions, the idea for the Sail Through Cancer Foundation was born. We would continue discussing the subject in the weeks and months to follow, as I was becoming increasingly passionate about this cause.

We left Forney Cove, headed for Prisoner Harbor. We had several additional tasks to accomplish on this trip, including recharging the batteries, making water and approaching close enough to the mainland to receive Internet service so Sharon could pick up her email. The second goal was to partially circumnavigate Santa Cruz Island, checking out all the little anchorages along the way in search of a suitable location to anchor overnight. We wanted to try to get into Painted Cave, a huge cave reportedly large enough to accommodate a boat our size. We got an early start once we discovered that we had only very marginal communications with the Baja Ha-Ha fleet. Much of that fleet had already traveled as far south as Turtle Bay, and with the bulk of the fleet scheduled to arrive there later that day, they would all be out of radio range for good.

We had an interesting day, sticking our bow into more than half a dozen cozy little coves, any one of which would have been a great place for an overnight anchorage, some so small we would have had to deploy a stern anchor to keep from hitting the rocky shorelines. Alas, the access to Painted Cove was clogged with seaweed, and with a strong surge running, we couldn't have attempted to enter under any circumstances. We arrived at Prisoners Harbor mid-afternoon. We settled on this location to overnight because the wharf and shore looked very appealing. I could drop Sharon off at the pier and then anchor the dinghy off the beach and wade ashore. As it was off season, we decided to tie the dinghy to the pier instead, taking care to park it well out of the way, just in case any large vessels should appear and try to land. From the pier, we hiked up to the Conservation Society's little lookout building, which afforded a scenic view overlooking the harbor and housed an interesting exhibit about the history and natural features of the area.

While I was trying out the ham radio that night, I made contact with a fellow named Fermin, a really interesting guy whom I'd met on the radio earlier in the week. Fermin studied and sat for the exam five times before he passed. I really admired the dedication of someone who wanted a general class amateur radio license badly enough to work so hard to absorb the difficult technical material in his second language, one in which he was barely fluent.

After chatting for awhile, we switched to another frequency so we could monitor the conversation on the Southbound Ham Net from Mexico. That was an interesting conversation, as we listened

154

to them work an emergency with a boat that was 95 miles from the nearest town with a hospital, and attempting to transport a guest there who'd broken her wrist. It was impressive how quickly the radio network sprang into action and organized a doctor, transportation and a possible surgeon – everything the girl would need to receive treatment as fast as possible. When the emergency transmissions were over, Don Anderson came on with his weather forecast. He said that Santa Ana winds were predicted to be moderate, but with 35-to-45 mile per hour gusts below the canyons of Ventura and Los Angeles. The marine forecast was only predicting 10-to-15-knot winds south of the area of the wind-prone canyons and into Santa Monica Bay. Since I really trusted Don Anderson and was fresh from our experience with those devil winds below the canyons just three weeks earlier, we decided to leave the next day.

Back in Marina del Rey, we purchased a colorful red and white cruising spinnaker. We tried flying it a time or two without a sock to douse that big-as-a-six-story-building sail and we weren't very successful. After some research, I discovered there was a roller furling system for a cruising spinnaker that worked much like the roller furler for the jib. When we got the specifications for the Roll-Gen, I liked it best of the various options on the market, because it didn't require us to modify the sail to adapt that system to our boat. We did, however, have to move the spare jib halyard out about six inches from the mast to accommodate the swivel. We had previously bought a Catalina Mooring Coil from its inventor, Stan, a local and well-respected rigger in Marina del Rey. We'd gotten friendly with him as a result, and Sharon had even done some work for him, writing an article about his Catalina Mooring Coil, which she'd placed in a local magazine. Stan was the perfect guy to build the mast extension and do the installation.

Although we'd practiced with the spinnaker a few times in light air, now we were going to have the chance to use it on a long, downwind cruise. We had a lot of fun with it that day, although I had some trouble getting the sheets attached correctly at first. It was very cool sailing in 10-to-15-knot winds with the spinnaker deployed. We felt like big time sailors every time we successfully put that sail up.

On our next trip to Scottsdale we had scheduled one final garage sale. We finally loaded the last of the things that were going into storage and headed out in caravan fashion for Palm Springs, where we'd unload everything and return the truck. Surprisingly, we had very little remorse, perhaps even no remorse at all, when we left our house behind in the rear view mirror. We had totally adapted to life aboard *Last Resort* and all we could think about was getting back to her.

The realtor had been instructed to take the house off the market when the listing expired at the end of November and to start looking for a tenant. We were very hopeful that we could get it rented before too long, as we didn't want to be paying a mortgage and other expenses on an empty house.

At last, we were off to make *Last Resort* our full-time home. Shortly after arriving back aboard, we learned that one of our friends in Ensenada was experimenting with the idea of doing aerial photography using a remote control model airplane as a platform. We decided to sail back down to Ensenada in January to get some good aerial photography of *Last Resort* with her spinnaker flying. We had a delightful trip down the coast, even using the spinnaker on occasion.

The morning that we went out to do the aerial photography there was almost no wind. Spike thought that his model airplane was safe to fly in winds up to about 10 knots, which would have been ideal for our purposes. But since no wind had materialized, I came up with the idea of putting up the spinnaker and driving the boat in reverse to keep it full. I knew there would be a problem with the wake, but I thought we could airbrush that later if we had some good pictures. You can't imagine how ridiculous I felt backing up under full sail, spinnaker flying. When a couple of fishing boats passed by we all laughed out loud as we wondered what they must be thinking about these crazy *gringos*. By the end of the session, the wind finally cooperated and we got a whole series of outstanding aerial photographs. Several of the images have since been printed in various sailing publications.

156

Spike called his company Spy Cam Air and created a website to promote it. Unfortunately for Spike, the Mexican authorities misinterpreted his intentions and he had to shut down his website. But he's since met with the appropriate authorities and convinced them there was nothing illegal in his activities, so he's still conducting his aerial photography business, only under a different name. Last I heard he was in the process of creating a new website.

On January 17, 2008, we departed from Ensenada once again, taking the first step of a voyage that would ultimately find us entering Alaskan waters five months later.

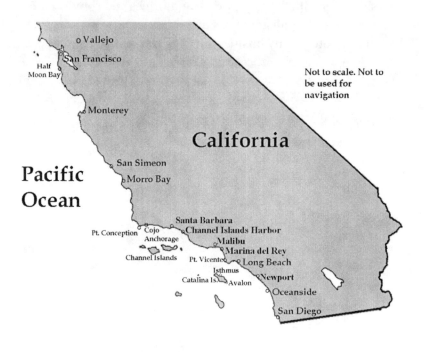

Ensenada, Mexico to San Francisco, California

Chapter 6

Ensenada to San Francisco

The first steps of our cruise to Alaska didn't have the feel of a long-range cruise at all. And really, they weren't. When we left Ensenada, we were headed for Marina del Rey to wrap up a few small things. Sharon was going to fly from Los Angeles to Germany to visit her daughter while I stayed behind to attend to boat matters. We also had to make a trip to Phoenix because we were due for our annual physical examinations. The doctors were watching a spot on my lung. I had one last round of scans before the doctors would either declare me cancer free or decide that it was cancer. If it was malignant, I would be faced with another round of treatments that would put our cruising on hold, perhaps permanently this time.

We were in no hurry anyway. Our number one rule as we sailed out of the Coral Hotel Marina this last time was that, no matter what, we were not going to be on a schedule, ours or anyone else's. From now on, our sailing would be dictated first and foremost by wind, weather and sea state, with particular deference to the tide and current, as we worked our way farther north.

We would be taking our time going up the coast. It was the middle of winter, and while Baja and Southern California enjoyed typical 60° F. and 70° F. days with moderate winds and seas, north of San Francisco winter storms were raging and the sea was a forbidding place upon which we had no desire to risk our lives. There would be no rush, and whenever we arrived in San Francisco, we'd plan on staying until at least mid-April. With the coming of summer, a stationary high pressure system, the Pacific high, sets in over the northern latitudes of the eastern Pacific, blocking the strong storms spawned in the Gulf of Alaska that regularly batter the Washington and Oregon coasts during the winter months.

With no real schedule, wanderlust our only guide, we decided to revisit the Coronado Islands our first night out. We had brisk winds on the nose and a challenging sail as we clawed our way north. The highlight of the day was spotting two gray whales not

100 feet off the port beam. Initially, it looked as though they were going to collide with us and as I contemplated what action to take, they sounded and swam right under the boat. They were content to continue on their lazy course in spite of our presence.

After a calm night at anchor, we were no sooner awake than we were rocked violently by the wake of another boat. When we went up to see who was stupid enough to be speeding through the anchorage, we discovered it was none other than a Mexican naval patrol boat. They were heading to the garrison on Coronado Island and I guess they wanted to take a closer look at us. Before we weighed anchor they buzzed us again, one and all giving us a friendly wave. I'm glad their curiosity didn't extend to an inspection by one of Mexico's legendary armed boarding parties.

We weren't underway more than five minutes when Sharon spotted another whale less than a mile away. We saw a 'whale' of another kind as we approached San Diego, for I'd spotted a nuclear submarine a couple of miles off the port bow, also headed towards the San Diego Bay channel entrance. We enjoyed watching a Navy security vessel and a Coast Guard harbor patrol boat take up positions to screen the submarine from any other vessels. At one point two Navy tugs pulled alongside the sub and one of them extended a boarding ladder, ultimately disembarking eight passengers. Meanwhile, the second tug attached lines to the submarine and began the process of ferrying it to the dock. At one point, Navy security thought we were a little too close, and they squawked at us to keep our distance. In spite of it all, there's something about watching our servicemen and women at work that gives you a lump in your throat. We couldn't have had a better welcome back to our home waters.

Once we cleared Customs, we went to the Southwestern Yacht Club, as we had on our previous trip, where we would stay for several days. We planned to be real tourists, so after dealing with a couple of maintenance items – the story of my life – we set off to the San Diego Maritime Museum. We explored a total of six ships, including the *Star of India* — the oldest and largest active sailing ship in the world (circa 1854), a Foxtrot Class Russian submarine, a very large San Francisco ferry boat — the *Berkeley*, and a couple of

160

other interesting boats. The museum itself is chock full of models, many of them warships from World Wars I and II, plus a number of photographs and artifacts from merchant marine and sailing ships dating back hundreds of years. It was a fascinating place, at which we spent almost five hours, but could have spent more.

The yacht club was packed with an overflow crowd and emotions were running high, because the San Diego Chargers were facing off against the New England Patriots in a playoff game. Sharon, who had gone shopping, got back too late to see the end of the game. That was just as well, because although the Chargers fought bravely, they were no match for the undefeated Patriots, and the mood in the yacht club quickly turned somber.

I had been talking to everyone who would listen about my idea to start the Sail Through Cancer Foundation and the response was encouraging. My personal story seemed to really be resonating, for while we were in San Diego, the editor of *Currents*, the newsletter of the Canadian-based Bluewater Cruising Association, called me to say they wanted to reprint the *Latitude 38* article that Richard had written. I had to track Richard down to obtain his consent to reprint the article, which he graciously granted. We had joined the Bluewater Cruising Association in January in anticipation of our trip to Alaska. This Canadian-based sailing organization has a membership of almost 500 sailors, many of whom have accomplished extensive coastwise cruising, ocean passages and even circumnavigations. We believed that by joining we would have access to a wealth of local knowledge that could prove useful.

As I talked with the editor, I mentioned our experience with the aerial photography in Mexico. She thought it would make a great cover for the coming edition, so I set about writing the accompanying story, which I forwarded with two of the new photographs. We were thrilled when one picture appeared on the cover of the March issue to accompany my cover story and the reprint from *Latitude 38*.

When we arrived at the San Diego Yacht Club, we learned that another friend of ours, Rick, had arrived aboard his sailboat, *Dolphina*, the same day, all the way from Cabo San Lucas. We mentioned to him that we were planning to tour the aircraft carrier

Midway and invited him along. We had a fascinating tour, even though we ran out of time before we could tour the bridge. They have actual jet fighter simulators aboard – the multi-million dollar kind, which you could ride for $8.00. They start you out by practicing on a computer for a half-hour. I guess they don't want you to totally crash the simulator. Being a pilot, albeit retired, I thought it might be easy, but believe me, it wasn't. I was able to keep the plane under control, but things happened fast and the dog fighting was really challenging. Sharon sat in the co-pilot seat and had quite the ride. At one point we had about six planes either chasing us or we were chasing them. One really difficult thing is not to shoot down friendly aircraft. The net result was that we got shot down twice after taking multiple gunfire hits on various parts of the plane. The simulator actually points straight down when you crash, leaving you dangling by your seat belt and shoulder harness until they can get it reset.

We left the next morning for the Oceanside Yacht Club. As soon as we passed the San Diego buoy it became clear that we were going to be able to set the spinnaker. It took a little while to get everything rigged, even in very light air, but by the time we reached Mission Bay the wind had filled in. We had a really close call off La Jolla. We were unaware that the kelp beds extended almost a mile out to sea and we had to do an emergency jibe in 15 knots of wind under full spinnaker to miss the kelp, which we skimmed for almost a half-mile before we were clear of it. Once clear of the kelp, I was able to adjust course and sail much closer to the rhumb line. The final spinnaker take-down occurred in 15-to-20-knot winds about 13 miles off Oceanside. All in all, we were able to sail 26 miles under spinnaker that day.

The guest dock at the Oceanside Yacht Club was luckily available. We were glad to be safely moored, because the forecast was for heavy rains. Not long after we registered at the club, the rains did start and it rained all night. The Harbormaster said we could occupy the guest dock without charge until the storm was over, which might be two or three days. We learned from this trip that on our northward travels, the idea of leaving port just before the arrival of a storm system might result in advantageous winds and conditions, provided we made port ahead of the actual weather front. This was one of the most valuable lessons we would use on our trip up the Pacific Coast.

We violated our own rule when we left Oceanside. Everything said we shouldn't go. Although there was a break between storms, the Thursday-night forecast for the next morning was for 15-to-25-knot winds with gusts to 30, rain and some squalls, even waterspouts and tornadoes. We were under pressure to go because we had signed up for a Safety-at-Sea Seminar at the Balboa Yacht Club starting Saturday morning. In addition, I had injured my hand during our emergency jibe coming up the coast off La Jolla, so I was hoping for an easy sail, not the forecast conditions.

When we left Oceanside, the seas were eight feet across the bar and they were so steep they looked like mountains. We had a rough departure, pounding heavily across three of these waves. Once out to sea, however, the seas were only about five feet with long-period swells, but as the day went on, the seas grew bigger and steeper. Only making about five knots and anxious to get into the shelter of Newport Harbor, we decided to motor-sail. We made very good time under power, but as we arrived the seas had reached such a state that we were literally surfing down the exposed channel entrance to Newport Harbor.

Our friend Shannon, whom we had met on Richard's catamaran, *Profligate*, had planned a dinner party at her home in our honor. She came to pick us up soon after we arrived and we enjoyed a lovely evening. She was excited to hear the plans I was formulating for the Sail Through Cancer Foundation and I credit her as the moving cause for the events that would lead me to this calling.

The Safety at Sea seminar was extremely well attended by over 100 people. It was a very informative seminar, reinforcing many of the decisions that I made when commissioning the boat, as well as pointing out a couple of deficiencies, most notably, our inability to adequately read the weather charts prepared by the Ocean Prediction Center. The weather portion of the seminar was presented by Lee Chesneau and we resolved to take a comprehensive weather class from Lee before we left San Francisco in the spring.

163

We were soon headed to Marina del Rey. Interestingly, President George Bush had been in Los Angeles and as we were sailing up the coast, we'd spotted a convoy of helicopters overhead. Abeam Los Angeles International Airport we noticed a Coast Guard vessel patrolling. Not long afterwards, we watched as Air Force One flew directly overhead at low altitude. No matter who the President is, it's always exciting to see Air Force One.

While Sharon was leaving from LAX, she planned to return from Germany to Phoenix. A week after she left, I drove across the desert to rendezvous with her. I was going to have a PET scan and was apprehensive about it. This test was going to be determinative as to whether or not the cancer had spread to my lungs. I was very nervous. When the test results came back, I received the good news that there was no change in the spot on my lungs. The doctors were now prepared to say it was probably scar tissue from pneumonia, which I'd had twice in my life, once as a child and once as an adult.

I also went to see my surgeon. He ran me through a series of tests and exams as well. At one point he indicated that I should raise my left arm for him. This arm was partially disabled due to the surgery on my neck and I wasn't supposed to be able to raise it higher than my shoulder. The doctor was stunned when I raised it straight up in the air, exclaiming "You can't do that!" When he examined me more closely, he determined that my body had compensated by strengthening other muscles in my back and shoulder, clearly the result of hauling lines and grinding sheets on the sailboat.

The last stop was with my family doctor for an annual physical. The results of the physical were also extremely positive. The maladies, including high cholesterol, high blood sugar and being overweight, that dogged me for years before I was diagnosed with cancer, were gone. My blood test, with the exception of a thyroid deficiency, looked as good as when I was in my twenties. All three doctors gave me a clean bill of health and their approval to fulfill the dream of cruising to faraway places. I was still afraid to fly, because each time I had in the past, my throat had swollen shut, requiring a hospital visit for a painful dilatation. But since the only

164

'flying' I planned to do was behind the mast with full sails that was a limitation I planned to defer worrying about.

I had found a wonderful solution to help me cope with living on a liquid diet. Carnation/Nestle makes a "very high calorie" version of their popular instant breakfast product, which contains all the nutrition and many times the minimum vitamins I need to lead a very healthy life. I had to pack at least a six-month supply on the boat for the trip, so we decided to order that in Scottsdale before we left and haul it back to Los Angeles in the car. Once the food was secured, we hit the highway for this final drive to Los Angeles.

One week later, all the provisioning was completed and *Last Resort* was ready to set sail again. We were watching the weather reports closely, planning to utilize our new strategy of departing just ahead of an approaching low pressure system. There was a big storm heading in from the northwest and it looked like we could get to the Channel Islands Harbor just ahead of it. The approaching front was providing favorable wind conditions, unlike the prevailing winds that would have been right on the nose, so on February 22, 2008, we decided to make a run for it.

As we sailed out of Marina del Rey, we both believed there would be no turning back. We really were cruising now and we both felt an initial pang as we struck out with no home but the hull around us. There'd be no home port with a welcoming slip to shelter us from the storm, nor the comforts of our now-rented Scottsdale home. Our ties to the land were cast off and we were vagabonds upon the temperamental sea.

We arrived in the Channel Islands Harbor just in the nick of time. We watched the leading edge of the storm front converging on us as we approached. We hadn't been safely tied to the guest dock at the Channel Islands Yacht Club more than an hour when the first winds hit — 35-knots with higher gusts that pinned us solidly to the dock while creating waves big enough to break completely over it, right there in the harbor. The day after the storm, our friends Neil and Eva drove up from Los Angeles to visit us. We all drove out to the jetty and were amazed to see that the remnants of the 20-to-30-foot seas the storm had generated in the Santa Barbara Channel were still big enough to completely engulf the outer breakwater protecting the harbor. A Coast Guard patrol boat was the only vessel to be seen, advising all traffic that the channel entrance was too dangerous to pass. Clearly, we weren't going anywhere for another couple of days. We ended up staying for four days waiting for the weather to settle again, during which we enjoyed the friendly hospitality at the Channel Islands Yacht Club. The dockmaster was content to let us stay as long as needed until it was safe to depart.

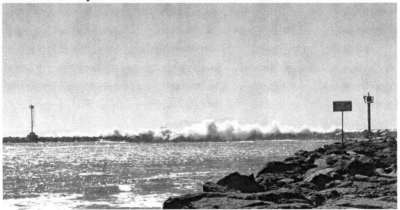

Two days after the storm, huge waves continue crowning Channel Islands Harbor breakwater.

When we finally did leave, heading for Santa Barbara, it was a beautiful clear day with ideal wind conditions, the kind of day that makes it all worthwhile. On a more serious note, we learned from the Santa Barbara Harbor Patrol office when we checked in that there had been an accident during the storm resulting in 20 people getting swept into the fence on the outer boardwalk when a huge wave topped the breakwater. The fence collapsed as the wave knocked three of them onto the rocks below, one sustaining a broken back. I was glad we'd decided to hunker down for a few extra days in the Channel Islands Harbor before leaving for Santa Barbara, despite our lack of progress.

Our first evening in Santa Barbara ended up being extremely interesting. Ever since first making acquaintance with Fermin over the ham radio the preceding fall, I had wanted to meet him in person. I had been quite impressed with his tenacity in passing the general class amateur radio license exam in his second language. He and his wife turned out to be lovely, warm people who both had engaging personalities. His wife was very petite, cute and was a live wire to boot. It turned out she was the full-time, live-in nanny and helper to an extremely well known political pundit and blogger. She had some incredible stories to tell, from this woman being too helpless to even fasten her own bra, to her callous treatment of her own mother. Apparently, as her mother lay dying upstairs where she'd collapsed in a closet, this celebrity and a nurse, who was called when the mother was stricken, drank cocktails downstairs. I don't know how accurate any of this was, but she spent the better part of the evening dissing this woman and could probably make a fortune writing a book of her own if she wanted. In any event, they were both delightful and truly entertaining company.

We were up at first light because we wanted to reach Cojo Anchorage in the lee of Point Conception before the winds became too strong. Sharon pointed out to me that it was "dawn," playfully defining the term, making a mockery of my fondness for sleeping late.

En route, I discovered there was no output from the alternator and, upon investigation, I discovered no power at all going to the regulator. The positive lead coming off the back side of the alternator was corroded completely through. I made quick work of the repair and replaced the ring fittings on the end of both wires leading from the alternator. I also discovered a loose motor mount, so I checked all the motor mounts once we'd anchored and allowed sufficient time for the motor to cool down.

It was a pretty roly-poly anchorage, but neither of us had the energy to deploy the flopper stopper. During winter, the prevailing swells are from the west, making all the west facing anchorages along the coast uncomfortable overnight anchorages. We shared the anchorage with *Mr. Clean III*, an oil clean-up vessel operated by Clean Seas along the central California coast. *Mr. Clean III* is a complete spill response system equipped with approximately 4,500 feet of boom, advanced oil recovery systems, high capacity stationary skimmers, storage tanks for recovered oil, forward looking infrared radar and advanced electronic equipment for directing and monitoring oil spill response activities. I would have loved to have a tour to see all the high-tech equipment, but it was dark by now and we had no energy to deploy the dinghy, even had we been able to finagle an invitation.

Before departing for Morro Bay the next morning, I contacted the Coast Guard to determine the conditions at the channel entrance. The entrance to Morro Bay is considered one of the 10 most dangerous inlets in the world, so sea condition, tide and weather must be heeded judiciously before attempting entry. The good news was that the Coast Guard advised us the seas were only running two-to-four feet at Morro Bay. Interestingly, while I was talking to the Coast Guard, they requested a complete float plan, asked us to call again when we left Cojo Anchorage and to check in by VHF when we were within radio range. That's the first time they'd done that – a pretty good service, I thought. It turned out to be an uneventful, almost boring trip and the forecast winds never materialized, which was a good thing since they would have been right on our nose. Sharon did see three whales while she was on watch and we saw several very cute sea otters just outside the harbor. Because the forecast included the possibility of gale force winds for the next couple of days, we checked ourselves into the Morro Bay Yacht Club until the following Monday.

The Morro Bay Yacht Club was having a dinner the night we arrived, so we joined them and visited with some very friendly folks. The first three people we talked to told us "I don't have a boat any more because I'm getting too old, but I have circumnavigated," "My husband and I built our boat and most recently sailed it to Hawaii and back" and "I just sailed down from Seattle." You don't seem to hear those types of conversations at the bars in Marina del Rey, where most of the sailors just voyage to Catalina and the other nearby harbors of Southern California.

Unfortunately, in the process of getting things ship-shape at the dock after we first landed at the Morro Bay Yacht Club, I'd re-injured my left hand, so I decided that when we reached Monterey, I was going to go to an emergency room and get an X-ray.

On Sunday, the weather forecast was for winds no more than 20 knots, so we decided to leave and only sail the short, 26 miles to

San Simeon. We had a real bum's rush getting off the dock because the yacht club was having a race and they wanted us to clear out immediately. We scurried around, only doing half the normal preparations and everything went smoothly until the current caught me and we started to drift into the outside boat which was rafted up in front of us. We grazed them, and while there was no damage to their boat, we later discovered a small scratch on our hull.

Leaving Morro Bay there were a couple of pretty steep six-foot waves in the channel entrance. We held our breath until we were sure they weren't going to break over our beam before we could negotiate the tight turn to seaward, when the waves would be safely in front of us. Once outside, we started to raise the mainsail, only to discover that the bottom batten had popped out of the pocket again, a persistent and annoying problem. We had to slow way down, lower the sail and attend to that in the heavy rolling seas in order to continue on our way.

I took some pain medication for my hand, which gave me a bad headache and made me nauseous, so I left Sharon in charge, with the LifeTag bracelet on her wrist as a precaution, and went to take a nap. When I woke up, we had a very nice seven-knot sail for the final reach into San Simeon. When we arrived we found one other boat – a slightly strange guy from Seward, Alaska, who was single-handing to Mexico. We were anchored in 20 feet of water, fairly close to shore, but even with the flopper stopper deployed, it was very uncomfortable.

In order to arrive in Monterey during daylight hours, we had to set sail at 3:30 a.m. It was pitch-black outside. About this moment I wasn't very happy with our neighbor from Seward. He wasn't running an anchor light or any other lights on his boat, so we had to maneuver around him using our radar. We never did see him in the dark, but we knew his position from the radar. It's very inconsiderate and pretty stupid, not to mention illegal, to anchor without showing the proper light.

We arrived in Monterey after a docile, 11-hour run up the coast. As we pulled in, we were hunting around for the fuel dock when a friendly fellow in a skiff came over to help us. In another 1400-

169

people story, it turned out he was in the process of buying a Catalina 470 himself and wanted to talk about our boat. Sometime later, when I went to check in at the office, I was surprised to find him there too. I found out he works for the marina, often in the office. We invited him down to have a good look at *Last Resort* and discuss some of the finer points to help him make his final decision. We learned that he subsequently bought a used Catalina 470.

Our first day in Monterey started with an early morning trip to a nearby urgent care center to have my hand examined. It looked to the doctor like a torn ligament because the X-Ray was clear. He taped my little finger to my index finger and suggested I rest it for several weeks. Clearly, he didn't understand the rigors of sailing a boat up the Pacific Coast, but I was diligent about keeping it taped and trying to protect it from further injury.

There was another important chore to attend to in Monterey. On more than one occasion, the 44-pound Lewmar Plow CQR anchor provided by the dealer had dragged, and I was becoming less confident in its ability to hold us securely in the conditions we would be facing as we headed farther and farther north. I had been told that the state-of-the-art anchor was the Manson Supreme. While it was expensive, I purchased one from West Marine in Monterey. I took our little rolling cart with me on the mile-plus walk to the store. I was stunned when I saw the size of the anchor and realized it wouldn't possibly fit in my flimsy little cart. One of the other customers happened to be the operator of a dive boat moored just two slips over from *Last Resort* and was gracious enough to load my new anchor in his pick-up truck and ferry me back to the marina.

I had an interesting mishap when I was installing the new anchor. The trouble started when I was trying to figure out what to do with the old CQR anchor. My first choice, to store it in one of the stern lockers, didn't work out when it wouldn't fit. I opted to try it on the small bow roller next to the one on which the new anchor was mounted, as theoretically, the system was designed to hold two anchors simultaneously. Wouldn't you know it? In the process the damned thing fell in the drink. We debated not getting it out at all, but then thought that leaving a $400.00 anchor on the sea floor seemed pretty stupid, so I had to bite the bullet and make arrangements for a diver to retrieve it, $85.00 later.

The day ended on a better note when we walked over to the wharf and had a lovely happy hour, followed by Sharon having dinner at the Monterey Peninsula Yacht Club. We finally made it to the Monterey Bay Aquarium the next day, where we spent a fascinating afternoon exploring and photographing the exhibits for my website. On the way back, Sharon got out of the cab a few blocks early so she could shop at Trader Joe's for some badly-needed provisions. One of the worst things that would happen to us occurred when Sharon showed up back at the boat limping, moaning and bleeding. On the way back from Trader Joe's she had tripped on some uneven pavement and took one hell of a fall. Now both of us would be nursing injuries for the balance of the trip to San Francisco.

After retrieving a shipment of mail, we made an early morning departure from the Monterey Marina. To our pleasant surprise, we were greeted by 15-knot winds off the beam as we entered Monterey Bay. The favorable winds didn't last and we ended up motor-sailing into 13-knot winds with one-half knot of current against us, delaying our projected arrival at Half Moon Bay. I was a little worried about depths in the harbor, as it was a very low tide when we arrived. At one point we only showed one foot of water under the keel.

It would be in Half Moon Bay where we would experience good fortune. The Half Moon Bay Yacht Club was having a spaghetti dinner that night, so I took Sharon there for dinner and an evening of socializing. During dinner, we met Stephanie, the club's membership director at the time. She turned out to be an enduring, dear friend and we would encounter her again on several occasions during our journey.

The sail to the St. Francis Yacht Club, where we planned to land after arriving in San Francisco, would be the final leg of this portion of the trip. We left at 7:30 a.m. to time our arrival with the current

171

while entering the San Francisco Bay, which put our ETA at the St. Francis shortly after noon.

This last leg of our voyage was not without incident. The 30-mile passage turned out to be the roughest we would encounter on the entire trip from Ensenada to San Francisco, and before long, we found ourselves pounding into steep five-to-six-foot seas. It didn't take long before we both realized we were taking way too much green water over the bow, which I immediately determined was the result of too much weight forward, with the new anchor now perched on the anchor roller. We had no choice but to heave to, so I could make my way to the foredeck and redistribute the weight while we were stopped. First, I moved the bag with the dinghy anchors back to the cockpit. We still had the old 35-pound CQR from the Catalina 36 stored in the bow anchor locker. As I thought about it, I realized that I'd never once used that anchor on the Catalina 36 and it was too small to be of any real use on this boat, so I promptly disconnected the chain and ejected it over the side. The boat immediately started riding a lot more comfortably.

Things got a little hair-raising coming into the shipping channel, because we almost had a close encounter of the wrong kind with an oil tanker, the *Energy Commander*. We were in thick fog, with almost no visibility, when this ship actually got close enough that we could hear her engines. A quick check of the radar and AIS showed the ship less than a quarter-mile off our port quarter, overtaking us as we both sailed in dense fog. I decided to check in with Vessel Traffic so they would be aware of our presence. As the fog cleared, we finally got our first glimpse of the *Energy Commander* off our port beam, less than 100 yards away.

As we approached the Golden Gate Bridge, we picked up the flood tide and made a fast transit of the shipping channel, at one point showing 9.5 knots speed-over-ground on our GPS – we were flying! As we sailed triumphantly under the Golden Gate the fog miraculously cleared, providing us with a breathtaking vista of the Bay, as the locals call it, before us. I snapped lots of pictures, including Sharon passing under the Gate for her first time.

It was March 8, 2008. We wanted to be sure the Pacific high pressure system was in full development over the North Pacific Ocean

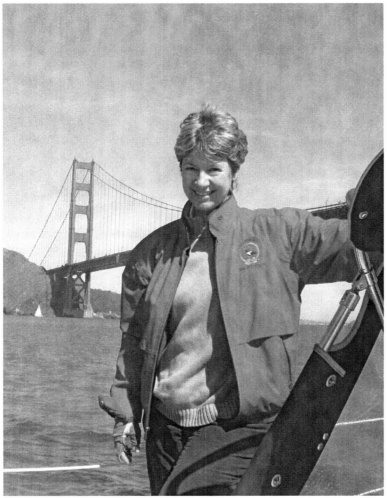

Sharon sees the Golden Gate Bridge from underneath, for the first time.

before venturing farther north, so San Francisco was going to be our home for awhile. The very worst 800 miles of the Pacific Coast still lay ahead of us.

173

Chapter 7

San Francisco Bay Area

Pulling up to the guest docks at the St. Francis Yacht Club in San Francisco, we were warmly greeted. There was a lot of action at the docks that day, with a major Spring Dinghy Regatta underway, plus an Encinal Yacht Club cruise-in.

Amy, the membership director, took time to show us around the club and came down to the boat later for a brief visit. We wandered up to the restaurant so Sharon could have lunch and lingered there to watch the dinghy races. They provided great entertainment as there were some spectacular wipe-outs, including a Flying Dutchman which capsized under full spinnaker right in front of the club. It was a photographer's dream, so I snapped away, getting some excellent shots for my website.

We left the St. Francis Yacht Club after a delightful week spent there. We had a fabulous sail to Sausalito, across the Bay on the Marin County peninsula, passing close to Alcatraz *en route* to the leeward side of Angel Island, followed by a vigorous beat to weather through Raccoon Strait, situated between Tiburon and Angel Island. When we emerged back into the Bay on the west side of the Strait, the winds were blowing over 20 knots, so the last part of the ride was really exciting. This was Sharon's first real sail on the San Francisco Bay, and it did not disappoint.

When we found our dock in Sausalito, a big catamaran parked near the end had tied his lines so far forward of his boat that there wasn't any way to get to the outer end of the dock. We had to pass to the shore side of him and the depth where we ultimately had to tie up was only three feet, measured from the bottom of our keel, at high tide, so I imagined by low tide in the morning, we'd be sinking our eight-foot keel deeply into the mud. We were getting pretty used to that, since one of our slips in Marina del Rey was very shallow and we had experienced the same condition. On our last haul-out before leaving, we had to paint the bottom two feet of the keel to cover up the mud stains. Not wanting to relive that experience, we prevailed upon the harbormaster to relocate us to deeper water.

I soon learned that our marina was less than a half-mile from the Army Corps of Engineer's working hydraulic model of the Bay. The Bay Model is a three-dimensional hydraulic model of San Francisco Bay and Delta areas capable of simulating tides and currents. The model is over 1.5 acres in size and represents an area from the Pacific Ocean to Sacramento and Stockton, including the San Francisco, San Pablo and Suisun bays and a portion of the Sacramento - San Joaquin Delta. During my years sailing the San Francisco Bay, especially when I was racing, I'd always wanted to see the model, but in those days it was only open to scientists and others doing research. We took the tour the next day. I was fascinated to learn all the different ebbs and flows within the Bay. If I were still racing, I'd have been over there with matchsticks to see first hand all the different currents on any given race course. As it was, I learned a lot about the flows and counter-flows outside of the Golden Gate Bridge, useful information for our departure later in the spring.

One of the main reasons for arriving in the Bay Area so far ahead of our scheduled departure was that a disproportionate number of my close friends from North Hollywood High School had settled in San Francisco. I was anxious to see all of them and was even organizing a mini-reunion of sorts, to have them all down to the boat. One of these friends, John, is a prominent marine biologist. When the Discovery Channel first started the "Shark Week" series, John could often be seen discussing his extensive research and knowledge about sharks. I wished that I could have coerced John and his wife, Pam, to join us in Alaska. His knowledge would have given us a unique insight unavailable to most, but alas, it was not to be.

Taking John and some other friends along, we had an exquisite day sail out of Sausalito and everyone enjoyed circumnavigating Angel Island. Shortly after leaving the dock and while underway, a sea gull landed on the dinghy. This was an unusual occurrence and we all managed to snap a number of photos before the bird finally took off, but only after hitching a long ride with us. Rain was forecast, which auspiciously delayed its soggy arrival long enough for us to get back to port.

Discussing my plans for the Sail Through Cancer Foundation with these friends was a big help in crystallizing my thoughts about how to organize it. After the *Latitude 38* article appeared the preceding summer, I received numerous emails from fellow cancer survivors who also wanted to follow their cruising dreams. Earlier that day we had a visit from one such person, Bob and his wife Mollie. Bob had survived throat cancer 20 years earlier and it had recurred. This time they were going to remove an entire section of his throat, including his voice box, and replace it with his own tissue. I know from talking to my doctors that this is a high risk operation, but I must say Bob was quite matter-of-fact about it and very optimistic about healing, eating normally and regaining some degree of speech. He seemed to find inspiration from my story and drove well over an hour each way to have the chance to meet me and talk about how I managed to get through it all. Bob and I have remained good friends and we keep tabs on each other's progress and health. Incidents such as these have been very rewarding to me and provided the motivation to continue toward the ultimate formation of the Sail Through Cancer Foundation.

From Sausalito, we had another lovely sail across the Bay to Pier 39. I had fond memories of Pier 39 and was anxious to visit there again. I had been trying for several weeks, without success, to secure a slip there. Some years earlier, the entire western basin of the marina had been overrun by seals, forcing the marina to close down all the slips. They'd built a series of new slips, but were still awaiting city approval to open them, exacerbating the severe shortage of mooring space. It had taken a visit and a personal appeal to the marina manager to secure a spot. I'd forgotten how strong the surge is in this marina and when we arrived, it was bad. I actually misjudged my two first approaches, the first because I couldn't readily identify our slip and the other due to the strong current. When we did put into the slip, we made a hard landing. Fortunately, the dock was well-lined with new padding, and no one was watching.

We had quite routinely assumed the role of tourists. Our second day at Pier 39, we hiked up to Coit Tower and took a number of the back routes and steep staircases that wind up Telegraph Hill. Lillie Hitchcock Coit, a philanthropist and admirer of the fire fighters at the 1906 earthquake fire, left funds to the city for beautification of San Francisco. Those funds were used for the construction of the 210-foot tall art deco Coit Tower. A series of murals, now protected as a historical treasure, can be viewed inside the first floor of the Coit Tower. These Diego Rivera-inspired murals were completed in 1933. It was a beautiful day for Coit Tower because the sky was clear and the visibility was almost unlimited. Hiking back down a different route, we kept hearing a commotion caused by a large number of birds, but we couldn't manage to spot them. We finally asked a couple of locals about it. They were quick to educate us about the wild red and green parrots of Telegraph Hill. While we were chatting, the flock flew immediately overhead and provided a thrilling sight. They are wild, self-sufficient creatures, and as anyone who visits this part of San Francisco will see, the flock is thriving. They are currently more than 200 strong.

It turned out that Vallejo, at the upper end of the San Pablo Bay, was the most convenient spot for many of my old friends to meet for a reunion dinner aboard *Last Resort*, so I'd made arrangements to dock at the Vallejo Yacht Club. Our prior attempt to use the spinnaker had ended in a messy dousing of the sail, when we'd suddenly found ourselves in 30-knot winds, so I was determined to haul it out and straighten out the rat's nest that remained during this trip. We had light, cooperative wind, and as anticipated, the spinnaker was a fouled up mess. In fact, it was such a disaster that I had to manually unfurl it, which took well over two hours and required a ton of work on the part of us both. We finally did get it flying successfully for awhile, until Sharon pointed out that I had the halyard wrapped around the headstay, which required lowering the sail while extended, dousing the whole thing and untangling that mess. We just managed to get the sail sorted out and properly stowed before it was time to turn up the Napa River towards our destination.

When we got to the Vallejo Yacht Club, we found the entrance too shallow to cross, so we had to hang off in the outer channel for about a half-hour, until the tide rose sufficiently to allow passage. When we finally entered the marina, it still wasn't fully high tide, but we were able to power through the soft silt. The sea level was going to drop three feet on the overnight low tide while we were there, so I was worried about damaging the rudder if we sunk too far into the mud. We would just have to see what transpired, as there were no options available to us at that point.

The highlight of our first day was when Dan, one of the fellow throat-cancer survivors who had emailed me as a result of the *Latitude 38* article, showed up for an unexpected visit. I was washing down the boat at the time, so I chatted with him as long as I could and made arrangements to meet later in the bar. We had a great time and really hit it off, wishing the visit didn't have to be so short.

The next day, after cleaning the boat most of the afternoon, we were ready for our dinner party, the mini-reunion of high school friends that had migrated from Los Angeles, who together made for quite a crowd on *Last Resort*. Unbelievably, two of the girls had their feet in walking casts. Combined with Sharon, who was just healing from her foot injury in Monterey, this made for quite a few nursing home jokes. At first we thought that getting my friend Barbara aboard was going to be a real challenge, since she'd arrived at low tide and the ramps were too steep for her to negotiate with her completely encased, injured foot. She didn't like my crazy idea of putting her in a dock cart and wheeling her down, but we finally found a second ramp that was far less steep and she was able to walk down slowly.

Inevitably, during the course of the evening, the conversation turned to my consideration of forming the Sail Through Cancer Foundation. The response I received from this group was overwhelming. Barbara, who has an illustrious public relations background and extensive experience working with charitable organizations, volunteered to do whatever she could to help. After that evening, my mind was made up that I should move forward with the idea and I resolved to give it my full attention when we returned to California in the fall.

179

All day I was worrying as the boat sank deeper, almost four feet into the soft mud, during an extreme low tide. While I knew the keel could take the pressure, I was growing increasingly concerned about pressure on the rudder. It especially scared me when, late that night, one of the Vallejo ferries, obviously speeding, created a large wake which easily penetrated the deteriorating seawall and sent us careening to and fro against the dock. I resolved to have a diver check the rudder integrity at the first opportunity. Having heard stories of other boats with large, exposed spade rudders losing them in heavy seas or from hitting an unseen object, we had previously purchased an emergency rudder, but the hope was to never need to deploy it, as is the case with all our safety gear. It would be an especially difficult and challenging task to mount the emergency rudder in conditions severe enough to snap the rudder post in the first place.

Our next stop was the Corinthian Yacht Club, situated in Tiburon. This venerable yacht club was founded in 1886. Many years before, while my Catalina 38 was in San Francisco, I'd attended a *Latitude 38* party there and had been sorely tempted to apply for membership at the time. Our friends Terri and Kimi were scheduled to join us for a ferry boat outing to explore Angel Island while we were there. I've said before that the best and most enduring part of cruising is the people you meet along the way. We had met Terri and Kimi during our ham radio classes in San Diego the preceding fall. These two are real adventurers, Terri being a pilot and both of them having worked for the National Outdoor Leadership School, which takes people of all ages on remote wilderness expeditions, teaching technical outdoor skills, leadership, and environmental ethics in some of the world's wildest and most awe-inspiring classrooms. The school maintains a fleet of Catalina 36 sailboats, like our old boat, in the Pacific Northwest and offers ocean sailing and sea-kayaking in one of their courses. After staying in San Diego for a time, Terri and Kimi had sailed their boat to San Francisco, where they would join us on numerous occasions.

The day of our Angel Island trip was the best weather we'd seen in some time. Terri couldn't make it due to a last minute problem at work, but Kimi was still planning to join us. It turned out the ferry

180

schedule was too infrequent during the winter to accommodate our plans, so we took *Last Resort* over instead. We were initially planning to hike around the Island, but as soon as we got there, I saw that they have Segway rentals. It didn't take me more than about two seconds to make a decision to treat us all to a Segway tour around the Island. We'd discussed doing something like this while we were still in the city, but Angel Island seemed like a far better venue to try them out. The ride was spectacular.

We were making quite the tour of the Bay Area yacht clubs and the Encinal Yacht Club in Alameda was our next stop. We'd met some very friendly people from this club when we first arrived at the St. Francis Yacht Club in the midst of their weekend cruise-in, and we were anxious to see them again, and get to know some of them better.

While we were moored in Alameda, Sharon left for a convention in Las Vegas. There was the usual long list of ship's business to attend to while Sharon was gone. I found a diver to change out the zincs, the sacrificial metal attached to strategic parts of the underside of the boat to protect the shaft and propeller, and to inspect the rudder. There didn't appear to be any rudder damage, which was a relief. Our satellite dish and FollowMeTV wasn't working well as we traveled farther north, so we decided it was time to bite the bullet and install a gyro-stabilized dish. I met with the local electronics dealer, and after deciding on a SeaTel unit and Dish Network receiver, mapped out the installation.

After riding the Segway on Angel Island, I became intrigued by the idea of having some mode of personal transportation aboard ship. After a little research, I quickly decided that the $6,000 - $7,000 price tag of a Segway was too expensive for us, not to mention that its 115-pound weight would have made it prohibitive to get aboard, at least without a lot of help from the electric winch. I was disappointed, but decided to keep researching what other options for personal transportation might be available. I had also learned of another personal transportation option, a GoPed® electric scooter. This scooter was rated to carry up to 400 pounds and promised a range of eight-to-12 miles. It was significantly less expensive than a Segway, around $1000.00, but with a bad knee left over from a skiing accident I'd suffered as a young man, I decided having the ability to travel more than a mile round-trip, my usual walking range, justified the expenditure. I'd found a dealer in San Francisco and when he called to tell me the scooter had arrived, I hurriedly took a cab to the BART station in Oakland and then rode the train into the city. This was a fairly new experience for me since the cities I'd lived in all my life didn't have commuter trains and I'd always had a car. After I picked up my scooter, I jumped back on BART and got off at the same station where I'd boarded in Oakland. Wasn't I surprised to realize I couldn't go back through the same tunnel to Alameda because there were no pedestrians or bicycles allowed? Apparently the ventilation system isn't good enough to support pedestrian traffic with all the car exhaust. Hence, the scooter got its first real test. It was over seven miles back to the boat, traveling a long distance to the first bridge I could cross. I had the scooter in economy mode, which I had to do anyway to break it in properly, and when I got back to the boat I still had about one-third battery life left. This was a watershed event for me, because suddenly I was fully mobile again.

The satellite installation took almost three days, but we were ecstatic with the results, not wanting to be without news and entertainment, especially since it was an election year, which promised to be very exciting and critically important, because the country was suffering through two long wars, a housing crisis and a looming recession.

As soon as Sharon returned, we headed over to South Beach Marina, a very popular spot, due to its prime location on the Embarcadero adjacent to the Giants' baseball stadium, AT&T Park. This is one of the newest stadiums in the league and we were treated to box seats, courtesy of our local friend Stephen, who would be joining us later in Alaska. We thoroughly enjoyed an exciting game against the Arizona Diamondbacks from the vantage point of these seats, right behind the Giants dugout in the Field Club section. We were big Diamondback fans in Scottsdale and were on hand for game six of the World Series the year they beat the New York Yankees for the championship.

Our new friend Stephanie, whom we'd been fortunate to meet at the Half Moon Bay Yacht Club, was joining us for a sail and an overnight visit while we were at the South Beach Yacht Club. Stephanie had a lot of friends in that yacht club, and as luck would have it, there was a big party there that night. Stephanie found my scooter quite humorous and apparently she will forever refer to me by the new nickname she coined, "Scooter Boy." After our day sail, Stephanie carted Sharon off to Costco, as we were beginning the process of provisioning the boat for the upcoming trip up the coast to the Strait of Juan de Fuca.

We returned to the Encinal Yacht Club after departing from the South Beach Marina. This visit had been planned to coincide with the Strictly Sail Boat Show, an annual event that we absolutely didn't want to miss. We wanted to buy any last-minute equipment that we might find on sale and attend Lee Chesneau's weather classes. We also had a surprise visit from our friends Norm and Charlene, who had shared cruises with us before, when we first took our boat to Mexico and later when we all sailed to Turtle Bay.

Lee Chesneau's weather classes were very technical, but provided us with the essential information we needed to interpret the Ocean Prediction Center weather maps available aboard, either through the Internet or by weatherfax, using the single sideband radio. Lee also confirmed a lingering concern I'd had about the GRIB weather files, ever since getting into trouble due to the conflicting weather reports I'd received in Turtle Bay. The GRIB files proved to be totally unreliable on that trip. Lee indicated that he doesn't have much faith in them either, because they represent raw computer data, unchecked and uncorrected by human hands. The second day of our weather class, we were introduced to the 500 millibar upper air charts, as well as the wind and sea state charts. The material was even more technical than the first day, but in hindsight, the information we learned was worth the price and served us extremely well while planning future passages.

Before we knew it, six weeks in the Bay Area had passed, and it was time to embark on the challenging leg up the rest of the Pacific Coast to the Inside Passage. Our friends at the St. Francis Yacht Club had agreed to let us dock there while we staged our final

183

departure. The night before we left, the weather forecast was predicting a large low pressure system, with a gale forming, to approach the coast within 24 hours. Using our newly-found weather knowledge and relying on the strategy I'd developed of riding the favorable winds generated by approaching lows, we decided to make a run for it.

We were filled with both trepidation and excitement about the voyage into the rough waters ahead, where like Captain Kirk, I'd never gone before. We pointed the bow seaward and sailed under the Golden Gate Bridge, downbound for our first stop, Bodega Bay.

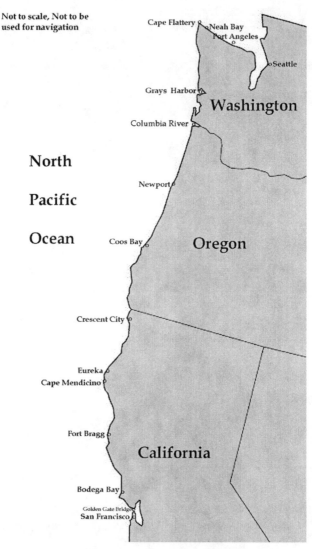

Not to scale, Not to be used for navigation

Cape Flattery
Neah Bay
Port Angeles
Seattle

Grays Harbor

Columbia River

Washington

North

Pacific

Ocean

Newport

Coos Bay

Oregon

Crescent City

Eureka
Cape Mendicino

Fort Bragg

California

Bodega Bay

Golden Gate Bridge
San Francisco

San Francisco, California to Port Angeles, Washington

Chapter 8
San Francisco to the Inside Passage

While on the voyage from San Francisco, until reaching the relative calm of the Inside Passage 800 miles away, we would be at the mercy of the weather and the currents. The Pacific high was just beginning to fill in as we were departing the San Francisco Bay Area and we were still vulnerable to the occasional fierce, late-season storm. Notwithstanding our successful completion of Lee Chesneau's weather courses, we still thought it would be prudent to retain the services of a professional weather router. We'd heard good things about Rick at Weather Guy in Hawaii. After several conversations with him, we'd decided to engage his services for this leg of the trip. His fees, based on a flat rate for each forecast, seemed more than reasonable. We asked him to provide us with daily weather forecasts and assist us with timing our passages, hoping to optimize the wind and sea conditions. If conditions were going to change while we were at sea, Rick would also email or call us on the satellite phone to alert us to any danger.

After consulting with Rick, we determined that we should leave earlier than originally planned, due to the rapidly approaching weather front. While the outgoing current wouldn't be optimal, Rick expressed his concern that we must arrive at Bodega Bay ahead of the front. As it turned out, we were swept out the Golden Gate at 9.4 knots on the back of the ebb and with some lucky timing, picked up the flood as we rounded Point Reyes, which helped keep our average speed at 8.2 knots. Those speeds meant that we should shave more than an hour off our time *en route*, completing the entire trip in just over six hours.

We arrived at Bodega Bay just ahead of the cold front. While it carried a lot of rain, the winds were far milder than predicted. Rick was advising us that after the front passed we would have favorable weather for the next leg of the trip to Fort Bragg, 90 miles distant, so we resolved to catch some sleep and leave after only 10 hours in port.

Alfred Hitchcock immortalized Bodega Bay in his thriller movie, *The Birds*. None of the original buildings from the movie have been preserved. What could have been a good tourist draw is gone. It turned out there was some local excitement when we arrived and it seemed the entire town had turned out to watch a beached power-boat being hauled off the rocks. The wreck of this boat on the breakwater the weekend before was the talk of the town and all anyone could talk about during our short stay, speculation being that the skipper had been intoxicated at the time of the mishap.

Planning passages along the northern Pacific Coast of the United States is much like playing with a Rubic's cube and often, just as frustrating. Currents at the departure and destination ports have to be timed to coincide with the end of the flood tide. Arrivals have to be timed for daylight hours. We didn't want to cross dangerous, unfamiliar bars while fighting a current or in darkness. All of this information was calculated on a large spreadsheet that I had developed while we were in San Francisco. As an additional safety factor, I had reenlisted my friend Norm to track our progress. Nobody would know our whereabouts and we thought somebody capable of notifying the Coast Guard should be in touch with us in case we failed to arrive at our various destinations. That meant sending him an email or calling him upon departure from each harbor and upon arrival at our destination, although I often sent him progress reports as the sea conditions grew more treacherous with our northward progress.

The entrance to Spuds Harbor Marina consisted of a two-mile long winding channel, which meandered through a maze of day beacons and lighted buoys, extending from the mouth of Bodega Bay to the relative safety of the marina. We were concerned about departing in total darkness, but given the weather and tidal forecasts, we had little choice but to shove off at 1:15 a.m. With Sharon on deck holding a big lantern, while I was stationed at the helm with my eyes glued to the chartplotter, we cautiously picked our way along from buoy to buoy until we safely departed the harbor and headed north once again.

188

The night passed quickly. I was somewhat amazed that we still had consistent Internet access with our Verizon Aircard, especially since it lasted this entire leg. By 10:00 a.m., we were three hours from Fort Bragg, when I began getting pretty nervous about entering the harbor. Depths are questionable and seas in the channel entrance can be very dangerous, so I called the Coast Guard to inquire about current conditions. Although they reported all was relatively calm, they still volunteered to send an escort boat out if we wanted. That sounded ominous. With good visibility and calm seas, we thanked them but thought we would be fine on our own.

It was a scary approach, with outcrops of rocks lining the way, but once we were out of the surf the depths were more than adequate and we didn't encounter any problems. Entering the Noyo River under the highway bridge was like landing in wonderland, a cross between a Maine fishing village and Disney World. We were so busy snapping pictures we forgot all about rigging the fenders and mooring lines and had to scurry at the end.

The following morning we hopped on a restored train that chugged through tunnels, over bridges and past open meadows, winding its way deep into a redwood forest, following the coastal "Redwood Route" as it has since 1885. Called the Skunk Train, a loquacious conductor told us all about the early days, when this train was the logical vehicle for moving massive redwood logs to Mendocino Coast sawmills from the rugged back country. We enjoyed spectacular mountain scenery already beginning to reveal its summer bloom, much different than the seascapes to which we were accustomed. On the return trip we were very relaxed and the clickety-clack of the wheels rolling along the old tracks quickly lulled us both to sleep.

We left Fort Bragg, again in the dead of night. Leaving this quaint riverside town, with its balmy weather and fragrance of spring flowers coming into bloom, made us resolve to spend more time here on the return trip.

We still had almost 600 miles of rough water to cover before we could duck into the comparative shelter of the Strait of Juan de Fuca. As there was no other vessel traffic in sight, we had the ocean

189

to ourselves. We were soon cruising in over 500 feet of water, well beyond the crab-pot danger zone

While we were in port, we had sought information from the local fisherman about rounding Cape Mendocino. Much the same strategy is employed by the locals when rounding this cape as we used to round Point Conception. The local fishermen usually anchor overnight in Shelter Cove, 32 miles south of Cape Mendocino, both to break up the long trip and allow for an early morning rounding. Since we'd left during the night and planned to push on all the way to Eureka, after confirming with Rick, our weatherman, that we still had a good weather window, we pushed on and rounded Cape Mendocino on this leg. True to reputation, it dished out some choppy four-to-six foot seas right on our nose. Lee Chesneau had emphasized more than once during class that wind and current accelerate around a headland, explaining the notorious reputations of Point Conception and Cape Mendocino. Almost immediately after rounding the cape, the currents, winds and seas eased, making for a smooth sail into the harbor in Humboldt Bay.

Eureka, the town at the head of Humboldt Bay, is known for its Victorian architecture, particularly the Carson Mansion. When I think of Victorian architecture, I think of elaborate bow windows, towers, gingerbread trim, wrap-around porches, odd shapes and unusual roof lines that are Carson Mansion hallmarks. We were assigned a spot in the marina directly across the channel, letting our imaginations fill with images of the luxurious lifestyles enjoyed by the mining and timber barons of the day. This is said to be one of the most photographed houses in California, if not the U.S.

Since we had just completed our intensive weather seminar, we were excited to visit the last California-based National Weather Service office. We introduced ourselves to the chief meteorologist on duty and another forecaster who graciously greeted us when we arrived. They were happy to show us some of the highly complex and sophisticated technology they use to track weather systems and make predictions. We were very impressed by the high-tech graphic tools they have available to aid their forecasting. They also confirmed what Rick had told us about the impending weather. We were going to have calm seas and favorable winds for a few days, but four days out there was real trouble in the forecast, with predictions of 14-to-20 foot seas and 30-to-40-knot winds. Based on that forecast, we decided to push on immediately, all the way to Coos Bay, where we needed to arrive ahead of the storm.

Notwithstanding the urgency to make a timely departure, we were forced to delay a short while to make a sail repair. On several occasions, our mainsail's lower batten had slipped out of its pocket and the various temporary repairs we'd made had proved unsuccessful. Finally, we installed a small screw through the plastic pocket and planned to test this latest short-term fix while underway.

As was becoming our 'norm,' Sharon slept at night during relatively calm passages, and this one would be no different. I managed a short nap in the morning, and when I awoke, I found the XO working away on her computer, in between watching the radar and keeping a look out. We continued to have remarkably reliable Internet connectivity using our Aircards.

When we arrived in Crescent City we stopped at the fuel dock and topped off the tanks. Between the engine, generator and diesel heater, we were only burning about a gallon and a half of diesel an hour, which I considered to be excellent fuel consumption.

Crescent City is one of the few harbors along the northern Pacific Coast that doesn't have an entrance bar formed by a river's outflow. It was nice not to have to go through the mathematical exercise of timing the flood tide to coincide with daylight for our arrival.

Crescent City is near the Redwood National Park, which protects 37 miles of rugged California coastline and is home to the tallest trees in the world. While I wanted to rent a car and drive over for a day, I also was anxious to continue our northward progress during this weather window. We were growing more excited each day as we got closer to the sheltered waters of the Inside Passage. We did make time to visit a big festival going on at the marina the day we arrived. We strolled around listening to live music, inspecting the wares of the vendors and watching children play the carny games. We enjoyed seeing the wood carving of the mermaid that watches over the harbor and stares intently at all passers-by, her long hair flowing like the sea itself.

Determined to push on, we planned another middle-of-the-night departure to start the next 115-mile leg. I was beginning to feel like a fugitive, leaving all these harbors under cover of darkness. We never encountered another vessel when leaving port in the dead of night.

As we departed Crescent City, several omens hinted at the ill events that would soon follow. The quickly building seas and winds were a clear indication that the forecast weather front was rapidly approaching the coast. In an attempt to engage the radar in the pitch black darkness, we'd accidentally hit the wrong button, and turned off the chartplotter entirely. Blind in the dark, I suddenly found myself disoriented and confused by the channel markers as we headed out into rough, six-foot seas. Things returned to normal once the chartplotter was reactivated. At 1:00 a.m., Sharon went back to the aft cabin to lie down for the night. I was wearing my LifeTag and monitoring conditions from the navigation station, occasionally popping my head out to confirm there was no shipping traffic. In the darkness, it wasn't possible to spot debris or seaweed in the water, so we just had to cross our fingers and pray when departing harbors late at night.

Not more than 20 minutes later, after Sharon had just dropped off to sleep, a screeching alarm sounded. At first I thought it was the LifeTag system, but quickly determined that wasn't the cause of the alarm. Seconds later, with an adrenalin rush, I discovered it was the high water alarm. My mother had a favorite term, "Grand Klong," which she whimsically described as "a sudden rush of shit to the heart." Well, just outside Crescent City, on this pitch black night in the heavy seas and strong winds, we had our own "Grand Klong."

The discovery of rapidly rising water in the bilge had shattered my usual confident demeanor. After tearing into several suspect locations, I remembered the problem we'd previously encountered with the shaft seal system, so I hurriedly opened the cover to the back of the engine to reveal the propeller shaft. Sure enough, water was flooding in. You read in Chapter 1 of my desperate calls to

192

Sharon, "Wake up, wake up." Somehow, she had managed to hear my calls over the drone of the engine and the howling wind. With my hands still trembling from the sudden rush of adrenalin, I enlisted her to help me tighten the small set-screws with the hex wrench of the proper size I had purchased from Sears after the first incidence of this problem had occurred in Mexico. Thank goodness I'd hunted that tool down, despite the difficulties in locating such an oddball size. Later, I installed a hose clamp on the shaft forward of the wheel to prevent it from sliding forward and breaking the seal again. We decided then and there to replace the whole system during our next haul-out.

In her writing, Sharon has a whimsical way of reinforcing the theory that men are from Mars and women are from Venus, as suggested recently in the popular book of the same name. Here is what she subsequently wrote in an article describing our trip up the coast from San Francisco:

Dick's hand is shaking too much for him to unscrew the bolts to the seal that was supposed to provide a water-tight connection between our sailboat's engine and the propeller. Sea water is gushing in around the coupling like the return of the Red Sea after Moses led out the Israelites. The piercing, electronic bleeping of the high-water alarm is incessant. As I shake off sleep and try to focus, one thought lights up in my brain like an old-fashioned burlesque marquee: What are two almost-senior citizens doing here, anyway?

At this point, I'm an unlikely candidate to master any Zen-like moments of spiritual calm. But, somehow, I manage to get the hex wrench started. In a matter of moments Dick regains his composure. He takes over again. I take a look at myself in a new light. Who is this cool-headed woman methodically reviewing a checklist of emergency procedures?

1) Finish getting dressed in the warmest clothes available (it's 2:00 a.m. and we're six miles out to sea – west, northwest of Crescent City, CA). Check.
2) Throw go-bags into our dinghy. Check.

193

Well, that's about it, actually. My other mental checklist is of items to do if/when we survive:

1) Enhance my list of emergency procedures.

2) Start drilling on emergency procedures.

3) Drill some more on emergency procedures.

Dick is now confident. He's reattached the coupling and the bilge pump has taken care of the excess water. This is like being married to Lewis and Clark. Let's face it, I'm living *his* dream. Apparently that dream requires extreme tests of stamina, endurance and nerves. We're pounding into scary-looking seas. My hair has been permanently rearranged into a charming monk-like coif from being anchored under caps to protect against 25-knot apparent winds on the nose. We're striving to beat our way toward the Inside Passage between Canada's mainland and the protective islands toward Alaska. Here's Dick's note from the log that day:

"APRIL 27, 2008 (SUNDAY): CRESCENT CITY, CA TO CHARLESTON HARBOR, COOS BAY, OR:

"Sky Condition: Overcast w/morning fog; visibility <1 NM

Temperature: 48° - 50° F

Wind Direction: N to SW

Wind Speed: 15 - 20 knots

Wave Height: 6 feet

Total Miles: 116.3. NM

Miles Under Power: 116.3 NM (Motor-sailing)

Average Speed: 7.25 Knots

"This will be the last very long leg for awhile. We will hunker down in Coos Bay until at least Thursday, maybe Friday. Six miles out of port an alarm went off. I thought it was the LifeTag, but quickly determined that wasn't the problem. Seconds later I discovered it was the HIGH WATER ALARM.

"It turned out that the set screws on the shaft for the PSS system were loose and the restraining wheel had slipped up the shaft again, causing a

194

flood. THE GREAT NEWS IN ALL THIS IS THAT OUR SAFETY SYSTEMS WORKED PERFECTLY. This was the first real test of the High Water Alarm. Without it, the floorboards could have been awash and the batteries shorted out before I knew we had a problem. After that, things calmed down, Sharon went back to bed and I'm answering a few emails and keeping occupied."

Now, does that sound at all like we faced down death in a scene that could be spliced into the film "Victory at Sea"? Does it even sound like we're on the same boat? I had no idea there was any *great* news, other than the fact we survived. Dick and I are living in strange and often complex, parallel universes. He's Peter Pan, I'm the conservative and reluctant Wendy. Or maybe he's Captain Kirk – going where no man has gone before – but hell, I'm still Wendy.

At 3:30 a.m. that night we passed a major milestone, passing from California to Oregon waters. As I checked our course computer, I noted that we had almost exactly 12 hours to go to reach Coos Bay. Rick confirmed by Sailmail, which I accessed using the single sideband radio, what the onboard Sirius weather satellite system was telling me, building winds and seas that might clock to the west as the front approached. The cold front was going to pass over us *en route* to Coos Bay. I didn't want to tell 'Wendy', but I was watching with angst as the barometer rapidly fell.

By 6:00 a.m. I was hoping Sharon would wake up within the hour to relieve me. I hated to wake her up. She had been traumatized. Somehow, she'd calmed herself down enough to fall into a fitful sleep, despite the pounding we took all night. The weather this morning was terrible – thick, wet fog, almost like rain. At last, I heard Sharon stirring in the aft cabin. Sleeping had helped dispel her fear, so she readily took over the rest of the way until we were about an hour out.

The weather had deteriorated further while I slept, so I quickly called the Coos Bay Coast Guard to confirm that the bar was open. Our ETA had slipped a little, to 4:00 p.m., but we were still making good time and were a full two hours ahead of the originally projected arrival time. The skies grew darker and the wind started clocking to the south, as forecast. The seas were continuing to build. We held our breath and kept the sails trimmed. We sneaked into Charleston Harbor and hunkered down only seconds before the front closed in. After 16 hours, which included our near-catastrophe, we were secure and snug from the driving wind and rain that accompanied the storm.

Our friends, Ned and Bev, had driven over from Eugene, Oregon and came aboard for a delightful evening. The weather behind the storm was clear, crisp and beautiful. Ned was anxious to go sailing. Say no more! In four-to-six foot seas and winds gusting to 22 knots, we beat our way out of the harbor, but returned on a following sea. On this short sail we broke our current sailing speed record, achieving 9.2 knots. So many of our friends and relatives questioned our decision to embrace the cruising life that it was always gratifying when friends like Ned and Bev, and many others who actually experienced sailing aboard *Last Resort*, came to appreciate the joys of our lifestyle.

After Ned and Bev left the next day, the weather closed in again, so I took advantage of the down time to attend to some ship's duties, while Sharon puttered around with her chores. Still radiant after our wonderful visit with my old friends, we felt refreshed and headed on our way to the next stop, Newport, Oregon, about an 85-mile sail. Rick's weather report called for improving weather, although it was still rough when we left, with 10-to-11 foot seas. We hoped they would reduce to six-to-eight feet overnight, otherwise we might have a problem crossing the Newport bar. We had a nice sail with favorable winds. The seas did subside, barely making it possible to safely cross the Yakima River bar. As we pulled into Newport, Rick called on the cell phone to tell us that our weather window would close within 24 hours, stranding us in Newport for several days. We decided to get some sleep in Newport and leave right away for the Columbia River.

Leaving just at dark, we planned to take advantage of the 20-to-25-knot southerly winds that would build overnight. At around 9:30 p.m. on May 1, 2008, our luck ran out. About six miles offshore, we heard a loud shudder and our engine ground to a halt. I

196

restarted the engine with no problem, but the prop would not engage. We had clearly hit a crab pot and somehow the line and float had disabled our prop. Crab pots are a constant danger along the entire stretch of coastal waters from San Francisco to Cape Flattery. The cages that actually trap the crabs are set in very deep water and tethered to long lines with floats to keep them from sinking. They are virtually impossible to see at night and can quickly foul a prop. In severe cases, the resulting damage can open a large hole in the hull and the possibility of sinking is a real concern.

We were able to sail back to Newport before the wind died out. The Coast Guard wouldn't let us attempt to cross the bar under sail in the light winds and big seas, so we were forced to arrange for Vessel Assist to come out and tow us across the bar. We spent a restless night worrying how serious the damage to the prop, shaft and strut might have been. Fortunately, when the diver arrived in the morning, it turned out that the line on the crab pot had been effectively cut by the Shaft Shark line cutter, but not before the remaining line managed to seize our folding prop in the closed position, rendering it useless. The good news was that there was no other damage and with the lines cleared, we were good to go at our discretion.

After conferring further with Rick, we understood that the approaching front would result in some rough seas, but the initial wave didn't seem to be anything we couldn't handle, so we decided to go for it. The alternative was to stay in Newport for at least two more days and maybe longer. It looked like the farther north we could get the better our subsequent weather was going to be, so we decided to bypass the Columbia River and push on to Grays Harbor, only 40 miles farther to the north. The entire trip would take almost 24 hours, so as soon as the diver finished his work about midday, we headed out. This time, we planned to sail into very deep water, getting as far as 20 miles offshore, where we were sure not to snag any crab pots during the nighttime portion of the trip.

As we headed out, Rick predicted that the cold front would reach our position at about 3:00 a.m., with northerly winds of 20-to-25 knots behind it. The wind would build slowly, and to be

197

conservative, Rick said to plan on gusts up to 30 knots. Almost to the minute, the seas and winds began to build just as he'd forecast and we started taking a pretty severe beating. By the time Sharon arose in the morning it was very rough, and since I wasn't able to sleep, I stayed on watch with her. I was getting used to carrying on with very little sleep.

When we were within radio range, 25 miles outside Grays Harbor, we called the Coast Guard for a bar report. They weren't very reassuring and didn't want to predict what the conditions would be for our arrival approximately four hours later. Sharon and I started the mind game of plotting a course and calculating currents, in the event we had to push all the way on to the Strait of Juan de Fuca and Neah Bay. I wasn't looking forward to that prospect because I knew the conditions were deteriorating, and as such, our arrival at Grays Harbor ahead of the worst of the storm was becoming even more critical.

An hour out, I called the Coast Guard again. They said conditions had deteriorated further and the bar was now closed to vessels under 30 feet in length. I advised them we were going to come in. It was almost comical after that, because they radioed us at least every five minutes to check our position, our estimated arrival time at the bar and to ensure that we had our life jackets on and all safety equipment in place. They did everything but ask for our next of kin. When we did arrive, we confronted steep, six-to-eight foot seas across the bar. The sea was alive with cresting whitecaps. The Coast Guard had dispatched a large dredging vessel to the bar to monitor our progress and to help in case we needed assistance. Going through these conditions in *Last Resort* taught us a lot about our sturdy boat. I had enough experience with my prior Catalina yachts to know they were strong boats, but the unique, structural fiberglass grid bonded to our hull by the Catalina factory, gave me confidence that this boat was more than ready to meet the challenges of extended offshore cruising.

We were glad we arrived when we did, because the winds were ferocious by this time. We had a difficult time and quite a struggle tying up to the dock with the winds pushing us off. Once securely moored, we settled in contentedly as the winds gusted to 30 knots, exactly as Rick had forecast. Good old Rick!

It was several days before the storm system passed. Once it was safe to leave, we decided we could do so in the afternoon, for a change. I figured we could ride the flood out of the harbor, sail throughout the night and arrive in Neah Bay in the Strait of Juan de Fuca just after morning light. The water depths are quite shallow for a long way offshore as you approach Cape Flattery and the entrance to the Strait of Juan de Fuca, resulting in seas that can quickly heap up to dangerous heights. There is the added danger of crab pots in these shallow waters. By leaving during the day, it would be possible to use up a little extra time by heading farther offshore and standing well off during the portion of the trip that would be accomplished in darkness.

As advertised, this is the hardest leg of the journey. Having no faith in what were supposedly "crab-pot free lanes," we followed the advice of some local crab fisherman who told us they don't set their pots in more than 55 fathoms. We set a course to hug the 60 fathom line (about 15 miles offshore). Sure enough, it turned out to be a real blessing that we left early, because even at 60 fathoms the sea was littered with crab pots. We decided to get into some really deep water. When we were in 500 feet of water, it occurred to me that I could have made a joke that we hadn't seen any more crab pots, but then it was pitch dark outside, so we'd never see them anyway.

It reminded me of a story I heard years ago about a young fellow who took his lunch every day in Central Park in New York. For days, he'd watched another guy tearing up little bits of paper. When his curiosity got the best of him, he finally approached the fellow and asked him why he was tearing up the papers. When the surprising answer came back that he was doing it to keep away the elephants, he said "There aren't any elephants around here." Without so much as a blink, the guy said "See, it works!" That's how I was starting to feel about the crab pots, now that we were in over 80 fathoms of water.

The sea conditions were about as expected – winds were 15-to-20, with swells of six-to-eight feet, accompanied by wind waves of about four feet, creating combined seas of 10-to-12 feet, all of it right on the nose. Because we left so early, it was necessary to slow down in order not to arrive before dawn. With the crab pot situation, the decision was made to stay far offshore until first light. As a result, when daylight finally arrived we calculated our position to be 50 miles from Neah Bay. We didn't mind though, because we thought that once we turned towards the shoreline, we'd have the winds off the port beam and have a great sail.

I'd sent my buddy Norm a position update at midnight and spent a lot of time during the night responding to emails, since there was a good cell service, even far offshore. Sharon wanted me to help her with some research for an article she was writing, so I occupied my time through the night working on that a little bit, too. As conditions deteriorated, we started to pound, so I abandoned my Internet search and focused 100% of my attention to sailing and navigating.

Shortly after 4:00 a.m. I got my second wind as I turned us on a heading directly for the Strait of Juan de Fuca. It was still an hour until daylight, but according to the charts, we'd remain in very deep water for at least an hour after making the turn, so I wasn't too worried about crab pots. One thing I didn't anticipate was that as we approached the Strait, we'd be blanketed by Vancouver Island. Sailing into the lee of the island, the winds died to less than 10 knots, the large sea swells disappeared and we were only dealing with some residual two-to-three foot wind waves. With the sails up and flying fully, we motor-sailed through the home stretch, reaching Cape Flattery at 10:30 a.m.

After we made landfall in Neah Bay, I posted our position to Winlink. We'd recently discovered a service through which I could post position reports on a Google Earth map and create a link on my website. By now, we'd heard that literally hundreds of people were tracking our daily progress. It had become important to post our position reports in a timely manner so as not to worry anyone. I also emailed Norm and few other people, advising them of our safe arrival, before turning in around noon. Exhausted, I slept for almost 12 hours. At one point, I awoke for about six hours, then went back to bed and slept another five hours, for a total of 17

200

hours. The last two days of the trip up the coast really wore me out. I was in better shape than I'd been for probably 30 years, but I wasn't getting any younger and at 62, long days and nights at sea took their toll on me. We weren't planning on any more nighttime sailing for many months, until our return to San Francisco in the fall. For now, I was happy to be done with 100-to-150 mile passages, big seas, and strong headwinds.

The following afternoon, as soon as the tides were favorable, we pushed on to cover the last 55 miles to Port Angeles, in Washington. We would stay there for at least a week. We needed to get our mail, attend to paying bills and other personal business, as well as get the engine serviced and give the boat a thorough cleaning. The boat had performed well on the 850 mile trip from San Francisco, but it was time for a little tender loving care.

Our stay in Port Angeles was busy, but relaxing, since we didn't have to plan midnight departures and pull 12-hour watches anymore. What a relief. Both the diver and the mechanic I'd hired gave *Last Resort* a clean bill of health and we even had some company aboard for the first time since leaving Coos Bay, when Sharon's cousin Richard joined us for dinner.

Sharon wrote that she'd made an "inside passage" of her own by making it this far, but in truth, our journey along the Inside Passage was still ahead of us. Alaska lay 1250 miles due north.

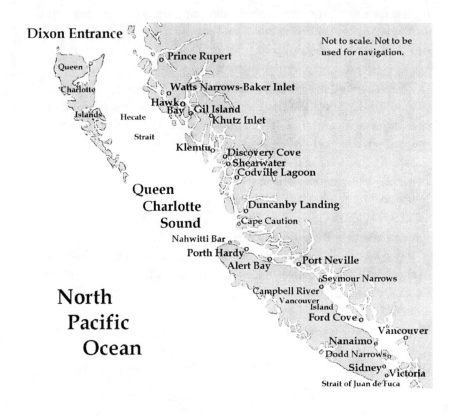

Dixon Entrance

Queen

Charlotte

Islands

Hecate

Strait

Prince Rupert

Not to scale. Not to be
used for navigation.

Watts Narrows-Baker Inlet

Hawk
Bay   Gil Island
       Khutz Inlet

Klemtu   Discovery Cove
          Shearwater
          Codville Lagoon

Queen
Charlotte
Sound

Duncanby Landing

Cape Caution

Nahwitti Bar

Porth Hardy

Alert Bay

North
Pacific
Ocean

Port Neville

Seymour Narrows

Campbell River

Vancouver
Island

Ford Cove

Vancouver

Nanaimo

Dodd Narrows

Sidney

Victoria

Strait of Juan de Fuca

Victoria, British Columbia to Alaska

Chapter 9
Alaska or Bust

We managed to accomplish all our chores in Port Angeles within four days. Our mail service had worked well while we were in the United States, so at this point I was hopeful our luck would continue as we moved farther from normal air routes. One constant challenge was keeping a sufficient supply of my canned food aboard. As I can only swallow liquids of a very specific viscosity, and then only with a substantial amount of sputtering and spitting, I have only found two products on which I can subsist. One comes in canned form and another in a powder that is blended with milk or water using our battery-operated blender. The canned food is easier to store and deal with underway, so while we were in Port Angeles, I ordered twenty cases. I made good use of the new electric scooter when the food arrived, because UPS dropped it off at the marina office, almost two blocks away. I made repeated trips with four cases at a time, but that sure beat making 20 trips hauling it in a dock cart on foot. The rides down the long, steep gangway to the dock, while weighed down, provided some excitement, but I managed not to drive into the frigid ocean water. Storage on any boat is an issue – there's never enough, but I managed do some 'creative' stowage by stuffing the cases and cans into enough nooks and crannies to get it all secured.

Because we had to be careful not to run afoul of the registration and sales tax laws of the State of Washington, we didn't want to remain in the state any longer than necessary, preferring to save our time for later, after our return from Alaska. We'd also started a discussion about the possibility of staying longer in the Pacific Northwest, possibly wintering over and sailing back the following year. At that point, it occurred to us that having exerted so much time and energy pounding up the Pacific Coast, simply staying for four months and then heading immediately back would be counterproductive. This meant we'd need to judiciously protect our travel dates to and from Washington so as not to overstay the prescribed time limits allowed for visitors.

We'd been in touch with our friends who lived in Gilbert, British Columbia, Bob and Nancy, a lovely couple we'd met many years before. Ever since my first cruising experience in the Pacific Northwest, I had wanted to return. When I first sailed here in the early Eighties, I fell in love with the area and was anxious to explore more, since I'd only whet my appetite. We'd originally met Bob and Nancy as the result of an email solicitation I'd sent to all the local yacht clubs trying to find someone interested in an exchange. Bob had responded. At the time, he owned a Catalina 30 and I still had the Catalina 36. After exchanging sailing resumes and getting to know each other, we both felt comfortable enough to organize a boat exchange. We spent two weeks aboard his boat cruising in the Gulf Islands and later they used our boat for a vacation in Los Angeles. We had plans to rendezvous with the two of them within two weeks of our arrival.

On May 9 we crossed the Strait of Juan de Fuca and entered Canada at Victoria, British Columbia. We discovered as we left Port Angeles that the bow thruster was inoperative, and with no time to make the repair, I decided it was something we could deal with later. I was surely hoping that we didn't find ourselves in any difficult docking situations until I could isolate the problem and effect repairs.

We were able to clear Canadian Customs with a simple phone call and were looking forward to our visit to the public wharf located directly in front of the world famous Empress Hotel. Unfortunately, unaccustomed to maneuvering in tight spots without the bow thruster as I was, I rammed the dingy into a piling, breaking a block on the davits and tearing a support ring out of the dinghy. I managed to jury-rig a temporary fix to the problem and while it would be easy enough to replace the block, it would require a professional to replace the support ring in the dinghy.

By now the primary elections were in full swing back in the States and I was beginning to have the time to really enjoy the new SeaTel satellite system. Senator Barack Obama was starting to give Senator Hillary Clinton a run for her money, challenging her front-runner position and presumed nomination as the Democratic candidate for President. The Republicans still had a host of candidates in the race, although it was looking more and more like Senator John McCain would be the winner, despite Governor Mike Huckabee's obstinate refusal to withdraw from the race until the last delegate was pledged.

Our stay in Victoria afforded me one of the first chances I'd had since leaving San Francisco to make good use of the new scooter. I was riding all over Victoria, from a long trip to West Marine for parts, to accompanying Sharon on her three-mile walks. Sharon tries to walk daily for exercise, so it was nice to finally be able to join her. We enjoyed a visit to the IMAX Theater in Victoria where we saw a film on over-fishing in the world's oceans.

The next stop was a visit to the Royal Victoria Yacht Club. *En route*, I had a flashback to my first trip to the area when I had been buddy-boating with my friends Virgil and Judy. We had taken a rather challenging shortcut between Victoria and Sidney on that trip, and as I looked at the chart, I remembered the spot, which we had promptly nicknamed the "Virgil Cut" in honor of my friend. Armed with a chartplotter this time, it was an easy matter to use the same shortcut again.

Our visit to this yacht club on our prior trip had been humorous. The Santa Monica Windjammers Yacht Club did not have reciprocity with the Royal Victoria Yacht Club, so only reluctantly had they allowed us to dine in the ladies' dining room, but not in the main dining room and bar area. In contrast, with our California Yacht Club membership and full reciprocity, they rolled out the red carpet for us. Sharon's birthday was the same night we stayed at the Royal Victoria Yacht Club, so while we could have dined at the club, I treated her to dinner in Oak Bay, at one of the better restaurants in the area. After dinner we stopped at the yacht club for drinks and met some of the members. Our primary objective was to attend the Bluewater Cruising Association's rendezvous and raft-up in Bedwell Harbour on Pender Island during our first full weekend in Canada.

While we were at the Royal Victoria Yacht Club I traced the problem with the bow thruster to a blown Perko on-off switch. With the help of one of the club members, and the use of their workshop, I crafted a small metal jumper to use while I awaited delivery of a larger, replacement switch. The repair worked perfectly, so the urgency to get the new switch passed. We decided to have it shipped to Bob and Nancy's house, since we planned to see them soon anyway. Bob had learned that the local Catalina dealer was sponsoring a Catalina Rendezvous, Canadian-style, the weekend after the Bluewater Cruising Association rendezvous. At this rate, we figured we'd be 'partying' all the way to Alaska.

Throughout the trip I had been inputting waypoints copied from the Douglass' series of cruising guides, published by Fine Edge Productions, to the Raymarine chartplotter. We had all six of the Douglass' guides and there were almost 2000 waypoints on our route of travel. Before leaving Marina del Rey, we had purchased a desktop computer for the boat. The laptop was too cumbersome and with all the computer-driven communications and navigation equipment on board, it only made sense to have a dedicated computer. Unfortunately, I couldn't find a system that ran on Windows XP, so I bought a Hewlett Packard Slimline that operated with Vista. Vista was an impossible solution. Few of the software vendors of the navigation and communications programs I needed had written drivers for Vista, so I had to either buy new software or get by in many cases using beta-test patches. But the bigger problem was that any time there was a power failure or electrical spike on board, Vista would crash the entire hard drive and I was repeatedly losing all the stored data. I backed up as often as possible, but still managed to lose a whole collection of photographs from San Francisco and other data. I also lost the Raymarine software that I used to input waypoints and which enabled me to transfer the waypoints later via a CF Card to the chartplotter. Without the computer to assist in this process, I was manually inputting waypoints to the unit, a tedious and time consuming project and one at which I worked furiously while trying to stay ahead of the demanding navigation challenges ahead.

We headed to Bedwell Harbour a couple of days early to meet up with Neil and Eva, other friends of ours we'd met in Mexico, who kept their boat in the Pacific Northwest year-round. They had decided to sell their boat and no sooner had we rendezvoused in Bedwell Harbour than they got a call to bring the boat back to the docks in Anacortes because the broker had a serious buyer. Since they were leaving, we decided to head over to the anchorage area and secure a good spot. We also had our first sighting of an adult bald eagle, which was a thrill for us. I managed to capture several good pictures, one of which was later published in *Latitude 38*.

The anchorage was moderately crowded, but I was constantly on the watch for power-boaters, who have a tendency to toss their anchors nearly on top of one another. Because sailboats and power-boats typically behave differently while at anchor, it is important to assure there will be sufficient swinging room before anchoring. What I didn't expect was for another sailboat, a Catalina 320 no less, to anchor too close. I squawked about it to the skipper, who seemed to have his hands full with a large contingency of guests aboard. He graciously said it wouldn't be a problem for him to tie a stern line to the shore.

Over the course of the weekend, we attended all the events sponsored by the Bluewater Cruising Association. We were very happy to find a number of members in attendance that had previously made the trip to Alaska and we gleaned an abundance of tips about the route and things that we must see while in the state. I thought we were getting our money's worth from our membership. The event had a significant turnout and at one point I stopped to photograph the sight of more than 50 dinghies lining the beach near the spot where the shore-side events took place.

Later, we took the dinghy over to meet the folks on the Catalina 320 who had seemed so ready to ensure we wouldn't be awakened by the sound of crunching fiberglass in the night. Kees (a Dutch name which he pronounces "Casey" in English) and his wife, Betty, turned out to be friendly and lots of fun. We found out they would be attending the Catalina Rendezvous the following weekend and we promised to get together.

Over the weekend, I received a phone call from Margaret, the back-country manager in Glacier Bay National Park. I was chagrined to learn that all the advance permits were taken for the period that Stephen and Katie were scheduled to visit, but Margaret said there are lots of cancellations and short notice permits are usually available, so we should manage. She also issued us a

207

permit for July 20 to July 26, so we would have plenty of opportunity to get into the Park at that time, when it might even be warmer.

As I've said before, the bane of any cruising sailor is to have to adhere to a schedule, but with Stephen and Katie arriving in Juneau on July 6, we now had to keep moving at a fair pace to cover the remaining 1200 miles. We left Bedwell Harbour and decided to put into Ganges, a small town not far from there. By now we had made the decision that if we could work out the logistics, we would spend the winter in Canada. Everyone told us the weather was quite 'mild,' so we set about trying to organize all the details. After learning of the challenges ahead and all the things there are to see to the north, we knew we didn't want to rush all the way to Alaska, only to have to leave again after a short stay in order to get back down the Pacific Coast before the end of September. We'd been to the little town of Sidney, located about 20 miles north of Victoria on Vancouver Island before, and remembered that the marina was lovely and first rate. In spite of being warned that it was unlikely we'd find any accommodations there, I've always believed in the theory that you never get anything you don't ask for. I called the Port Sidney Marina to inquire about renting a slip from October 1 through March 31, and much to my surprise, we were able to secure the last 50-foot slip they had available for the winter.

But alas, our good luck was about to run out again. Overnight in Ganges, our Webasto heater failed, and it seemed to be a fault with the combustion fan. I needed to get some technical support in the morning and then figure out how to get the unit back up and running as soon as possible. We simply couldn't travel to Alaska, even in the summer, without a functioning diesel heater. We learned that there was a Webasto dealer near our intended destination at the Port Sidney Marina, where we were going to look at our slip and sign the paperwork. We had more trouble *en route* when I noticed, once again, that the alternator wasn't producing electricity. I discovered that the same electrical wires I'd repaired once before were again badly corroded and frayed, so I reattached those two wires using new connectors and at least that problem was solved.

It was a lucky coincidence that we were going to Sidney anyway. In speaking with the Webasto technical support staff, I learned that they had a service outlet at the Van Isle Marina, so instead of going into the Port Sidney Marina, we diverted to nearby Tsehum Harbour. The local technician confirmed that the combustion fan had, indeed, burned out. It was going to take three to four weeks to get the heater shipped out for repair and back. The prospect of aborting our trip to Alaska wasn't an option. Reluctantly, I decided the best thing to do would be to buy a new replacement heater, ship the old one out for repair and retrieve it later as a backup. After dropping the dinghy off with another local repair shop to get the lifting ring that we'd damaged in Victoria fixed, we headed out to the Catalina Rendezvous.

By the time we arrived in Telegraph Harbour, there was a large contingency of Catalina sailboats already in the marina. Fortunately, they had reserved an outer end-tie for us, as we were the only Catalina 470, the largest boat in the fleet, scheduled to participate. We had a lovely sail from Sidney to Telegraph Harbour. The route requires passing through Sansum Narrows, a twisting channel where the currents can be strong enough to require diligence to the tide tables when planning a transit. At the northern end of the narrows, we had to pass under four, high-tension electric cables. With a 65-foot tall mast, I'm always nervous when going under bridges or other obstacles, but the chart said there was 150-foot clearance, so we forged ahead.

Telegraph Harbour was a lovely setting and we continued to be blessed with beautiful, warm weather and temperatures in the mid-seventies. We were wondering if our good fortune would hold as we headed north. We reconnected with Kees and Betty and made a lot of new friends at the Catalina Rendezvous. After the first full day we were feeling like rock stars. Most of the attendees had never seen a Catalina 470, so our day was filled with visitors wanting a tour of the boat. Many returned to our boat on Saturday night, several bringing guitars for an impromptu hootenanny, an appropriate continuation of the weekend's Sixties theme. Our cockpit overflowed with great people until the wee hours of the morning. In the end, we were very glad that we'd decided to delay our departure from the Gulf Islands long enough to attend. With our decision to winter in Sidney, it would surely be a blessing to have a small circle of friends, especially Betty and Kees, whose company we thoroughly enjoyed. The weekend seemed to fly by, and before we knew it, we were heading back to Sidney to arrange for installation of the new heater and to retrieve our patched-up dinghy.

En route back to Sidney, we received word that the heater had been delayed by customs, so we had an extra day. I'd heard a lot about Maple Bay, so we decided to put in there. As we approached the northern end of Sansum Narrows, something didn't look right to me. I know I'm paranoid about bridges and cables, but I could swear the electric lines were much lower than they'd been two days earlier when we'd passed. As we got closer, I was becoming increasingly alarmed and finally slowed the boat to a crawl. Sharon thought I was being silly, but when we were almost under them, I decided to head straight for shore, where the cables made a steep climb to the tower, thinking I'd have more clearance. As I sighted across the channel, it looked to me like the cables were lower than the top of the mast where they crossed center-channel. I couldn't understand it and was still pondering as we proceeded to tie up at the Maple Bay Yacht Club for the night. When I was checking in, the dockmaster inquired where we'd come from. When I told him we'd come from Telegraph Harbour to the north, he looked astonished. It was then that I learned the channel was supposed to have been closed to all traffic because they had lowered the cables to replace one and perform maintenance on the others. He said they had been broadcasting the closure on the VHF radio, but even with the diligent radio watch I always maintain, we never heard the notice to mariners announcing the closure. We were damn lucky, I suspect.

Within just a day of our arrival back in Sidney, the new heater was installed and the dinghy retrieved. We planned to test the heater overnight and resume our Alaska journey the following morning. While we'd enjoyed our social activities and all the new people we'd met in British Columbia, we were anxious to be on our way. We only had half the miles we needed to travel under our keel and Alaska beckoned. Our first stop would be the Nanaimo Yacht Club where we were going to meet our friend Bob. He had promised to bring the new switch for the bow thruster to us at the Catalina Rendezvous, but he hadn't been able to make it to the rendezvous because of high seas and strong winds in the Strait of Georgia. Bob was recovering from open heart surgery and didn't want to push himself beyond his limits.

The route from Sidney to Nanaimo meant two things. First, we had to retrace our steps under the power lines that cross Sansum Narrows, but more ominously, we needed to pass through Dodd Narrows. Years before, when I was on Bob's boat during our exchange, I had avoided Dodd Narrows. The prospect of eight-knot currents and dangerous eddies had convinced me I'd rather add 14 miles to the trip than risk it, especially in a borrowed boat. But if we were going to Alaska, we'd better get used to narrow channels with turbulent currents, so we laid in a course through Dodd Narrows and cast off. Fortunately, the power lines appeared to be back to their proper height and we passed under without concern. When we arrived at Dodd Narrows there were several boats hovering around the entrance, including a barge with a large tow. Bob had said to watch for tugs transiting the various narrows, because they only go at slack tide, so you can count on safe conditions if your timing is the same – a practice we would follow for the entire trip. I didn't want to be stuck behind the barge, however, and find myself with limited maneuvering room at a slow speed, so I pushed the throttle to 3400 rpm and sped off to overtake and pass the tug before we entered the restricted channel. We made it with ease and started to proceed through the narrows. This was not the time to be making mistakes, but I'd made a big one. Our diesel heater only draws fuel from one of our three tanks, so occasionally I have to transfer fuel between tanks to keep that one full. On the way to Dodd Narrows I had switched the valves to transfer fuel and in the excitement of passing the barge, totally forgotten about it. Before we could safely pass through the restricted channel the tank ran dry and the motor died. With a shout, I gave Sharon the wheel and raced below to switch the levers before the engine sucked in so much air that it would refuse to restart. As I passed hurriedly through the cockpit, I couldn't help noticing the swirling eddies developing just yards from our hull as the velocity of the current once again started to increase. Fortunately the engine restarted immediately and we continued through without incident, wondering all the while what the tug captain was thinking when we suddenly slowed dramatically at a particularly precarious point in our passage.

We were excited to see Bob when we arrived at the Nanaimo Yacht Club. Since I'd met him years before, he'd left his job at a local college to open a radio station. He was doing very well and was in Nanaimo working on the licensing for a second station. He came aboard and after delivering the new switch for the bow thruster and getting settled, we enjoyed a delightful afternoon catching up and enjoying the balmy weather which continued. However, Bob warned us that once we reached the upper half of Vancouver Island and entered Johnstone Strait, the weather would deteriorate and we might not see much sunshine from there north. I'd read stories of 80° F. and warmer weather in Alaska, so I gave little heed to his warning. After being kind enough to chauffeur us to the market and the local chandlery for last minute provisions, we enjoyed a lovely dinner aboard. We'd hoped to see Nancy, but that was going to have to wait until we returned in the fall.

By now we were becoming extremely anxious to be on our way, so early the next morning, after checking in with Barbara on the ham net and topping the fuel tanks, off we went, downbound for Alaska. From here on out, our daily runs would be much shorter than the 100-plus mile passages had been on the offshore portion of the trip, averaging only 40-to-50 miles a day. The excitement began soon after we departed. First, we had to clear the Whiskey-Golf Military Exercise Area, a torpedo test area into which private boats are not allowed while operations are being carried out. We'd heard on the VHF radio that the area was "active," meaning they were most likely firing live ammunition. Once we were able to navigate further from the shore and entered the open expanse of the Strait of Georgia, we saw our first pod of Orcas. At first, I didn't know what we were seeing. An Orca's fin at a distance could easily be mistaken for the periscope of a submarine. I thought there must be a submarine at work in the area. The people who monitor and look after the marine life in the Pacific Northwest are very well organized and we understood that they actually know and track every pod and individual Orca in the area. We would have more ominous encounters with Orcas during our travels in Alaska.

We stopped overnight at Ford Cove, near a thriving artists' colony on Hornby Island. There always seems to be some challenge to the boating life, and Ford Cove was no exception, because here we were confounded by there being 20-amp electrical outlets, which I'd never seen before and for which I didn't carry the proper adapter. We had to use our generator for power that night and vowed to find the appropriate adapter at the first chandlery we saw. The trip from Hornby Island to Campbell River would be one of the best sails we would enjoy since leaving the open ocean. The winds were from the south, so I set the whisker pole and we raced along, wing-on-wing. With the help of the current, we achieved speeds in excess of nine knots. Our speeds rivaled our record we'd set in Oregon.

We made a fast trip to the Discovery Marina in Campbell River, a busy fishing center. The resorts in the area are packed with anglers from all over the world during the season. We'd arrived a little before the start of the season so it wasn't too crowded yet. I wanted to try my hand at salmon fishing, so I set off to the local chandlery to buy a fishing license and the 20-amp adapter that I needed too. While there, I didn't find the adaptor, but I did learn of a fishing charter outfit and thought it might be a great idea to go with a guide my first time, so I could learn how to catch salmon from a pro. Salmon swim in very deep water, requiring fishing boats to use a down-rigger, not a piece of equipment that adapts easily to a sailboat, especially one with a Bimini top, an arch supporting four solar panels, an elaborate antenna array and a davit-mounted dinghy on the stern. Yes, going out on someone else's boat was for me, so I signed up for a four-hour charter the next morning.

We fished for over three hours and I never got a bite, but we did catch over ten pounds of prawns in the pot we set on our way to the salmon fishing grounds, so the trip was a success. I learned what I needed to know about salmon fishing and Sharon had a prawn feast for the next few days. We both liked the atmosphere

213

of Campbell River and pledged to visit the town again on the return trip.

The following day would bring one of the more serious tests of my ability to negotiate the trickier obstacles we would encounter in the Inside Passage and my navigation skills, for we would be transiting Seymour Narrows. These narrows present a formidable challenge, equally as dangerous as Dodd Narrows. While the channel is wide, the current here can reach speeds of 10 knots, easily overpowering a slow-moving boat, and dangerous whirlpools develop when the current is running that can totally engulf and swamp a boat our size. Many lives have been lost in Seymour Narrows. Years ago, Ribbon Rock was located mid-channel at the south end of the narrows and many ships were lost before the rock was removed as the result of a monumental engineering feat. Even so, for a boat our size, the hazards were still all too real. Fearful that my timing might be off, I had a fitful sleep that night. We arose at 4:45 a.m. so we could leave at first light. We ended up leaving too early, putting us at the narrows almost an hour before slack tide. We had to slow our progress as a result. Fortunately, a large, faster-moving tug boat towing a huge container barge soon overtook us. I was able to adjust our speed to time our passage with his. At slack tide, Seymour Narrows looked like a lily pond and I wondered what all the consternation had been about.

After exiting the narrows, we entered Johnstone Strait. I'd read much about this area and we were struck immediately by the change of scenery. Miles of towering mountains extend from the temperate, summer weather at sea level to the winter chill pierced by their snowy peaks. Along the shoreline there were no signs of man's encroachment. These pristine waters, although traveled day and night by cruise ships, fishermen and sailors like us, remained unattainable, refusing even a faint hint of the frequent intrusions. We were steadily approaching the desolate upper reaches of British Columbia. The sailing instructions contain frequent warnings of the dangerous waves that can heap up when the current opposes the wind. I had considered this in planning the day's route, with our intended destination at a small anchorage on Helmcken Island, well within reach before the next tide change. As we continued

214

through Johnstone Strait the winds were steadily building and soon we were motoring into 25 knot winds. When we reached Helmcken Island, we were dismayed to find another sailboat anchored, leaving no room for us to anchor with sufficient swinging room. We only had the options of back-tracking or pushing on to the next likely anchorage, Port Neville. We were of no mind to lose ground. As we pushed on, the tide started to change. Almost immediately, we found ourselves pounding over six-foot wind-driven waves. It was a wet, uncomfortable ride. We always motor with our mainsail up, but this time the sail was flogging wildly. Afraid of tearing it or dislodging one of the battens again, I opted to lower the sail. I was too late. One of the batten pockets fell off completely before I could get the sail down. The hour it took to reach Port Neville seemed like an eternity and we were never happier to drop our anchor and retreat to the warm shelter of our cozy cabin as the winds howled outside.

Our next stop was Alert Bay where we found a gem, the U'mista Cultural Centre, one of the longest-operating and most successful First Nations cultural facilities in British Columbia. It was founded in 1980 as a ground breaking project to house potlatch artifacts which had been seized by the Canadian government during an earlier period of cultural repression. The return of the potlatch artifacts not only provided U'mista's name ("the return of something important"), but sparked a general trend toward repatriation of First Nations cultural artifacts. It prompted the creation of a physical facility and human resources infrastructure, which have continued to successfully operate for over two decades. Alert Bay is supposed to be a place where the Orcas pull right up to the beach to attack seals or scratch their bellies. Now we have an excuse to return, since we didn't see any Orcas while there.

From Alert Bay we headed to Port Hardy. When we called the marina we were very disappointed to learn there was no room until the following day. We now had two priorities, first and foremost to repair the sail, and second, to receive a shipment of mail. We had no choice but to moor overnight at the public docks which are frequented by fishing boats. I have no quarrel with fishermen, but because they have to keep their catch alive, they run their gen-

215

erators all night, a noisy, smelly proposition that doesn't lend itself to a good night's rest. We were happy to receive a radio call from the marina first thing in the morning that they had a spot for us. Port Hardy is a town of several thousand people and we'd planned to stay three days, which I'd hoped would be long enough for the mail to arrive. To fix the batten pocket I drilled two holes through the plastic pocket holders on both sides of the mainsail, while drilling through the batten itself, and the sail. I then used large fender washers and through-bolted the whole arrangements. That ought to hold it, I thought.

The weather was horrible and we found ourselves stuck in Port Hardy much longer than we had planned. While there, we briefly met Christy and Bucky on the motor vessel "Un-Doc'd." They would play a big role in our lives that summer. The mail arrived, but a suitable weather window for Crossing Queen Charlotte Sound still eluded us. The Inside Passage consists almost entirely of protected waters, but between Victoria and Alaska there are two notorious stretches of open ocean, Queen Charlotte Sound and Dixon Entrance. We were about to experience the former. As we impatiently waited for our first opportunity to leave Port Hardy, I spent my time studying the charts and the prevailing weather. I was formulating a strategy for the crossing. If we took the standard route, we would head in a northwesterly direction that would put the winds right on our nose as we rounded aptly-named Cape Caution. But what if we risked crossing the Nahwitti Bar and departed from Port Hardy on a more westerly course before crossing Queen Charlotte Sound? It was possible that such a plan would put us on a reach, the safest and most comfortable point of sail, as we dealt with the 12-foot seas and 15-to-20 knot winds that were forecast for Queen Charlotte Sound. The sailing instructions describe breaking waves across the Nahwitti Bar, which shallows suddenly to only 30 feet, causing the seas to build up dangerously, often actually breaking. While our forecast included big seas, the wind wasn't supposed to build until afternoon, so we settled on this strategy and shoved off, emboldened by our previously successful passages through both Dodd and Seymour narrows.

Because we'd left very early to time our arrival at the bar with slack tide, Sharon thought she'd take a nap before we arrived there. When I neared the bar, the accuracy of the tide tables was clearly questionable. There were steep waves and they were breaking in places. This was going to be one wild ride. Halfway across the bar Sharon flew into the cockpit, inquiring groggily what was going on. I was holding the wheel for dear life as we pounded heavily over what appeared to be near-vertical standing waves. It was a rough few minutes, but the decision paid off. When we turned toward Rivers Inlet, the seas, while large, were long-period and rolled gently under our beam as we got a thrill from the brisk five-hour sail across Queen Charlotte Sound. Another of the storied hurdles was behind us.

I have always liked to gunkhole and this day would be no exception. We were headed for Duncanby Landing, an exclusive fishing resort in Goose Bay, six miles up the channel from the entrance to Rivers Inlet. As we passed, I was intrigued by the numerous islets that dotted the shoreline along the route to the main entrance to Goose Bay. It looked to me that if one was careful, a nice shortcut could be found between these scenic islets. After consulting with Sharon, we decided to go for it. At first I put her on the bow to watch for uncharted rocks, which we'd been repeatedly told were a constant hazard in these waters – including by our agent, as he sheepishly explained away the expensive surcharge demanded by our insurance carrier for this trip. When it was obvious the visibility was too poor to be able to see a rock lurking even just a few feet below the surface, I called the XO back to the cockpit and tasked her to keep her eyes glued to the depth sounder. As I was threading my way through a maze of islets and rocks awash, Sharon suddenly started frantically calling out rapidly-declining depths. I threw the engine into full reverse and finally brought the shuddering boat to a dead stop with only one foot of water remaining under the keel, a dangerously close call. We proceeded on at dead slow until we successfully navigated the meandering channels and were in the deep, open waters of Goose Bay. Duncanby Landing was still deserted and we enjoyed the solitude as we set off for a hike along the creek that led into the mountains behind the newly-remodeled lodge, which now sported new, bright red roofs.

We would soon find that the scenery was only going to get better. The Codville Lagoon Marine Sanctuary is virtually hidden from Fisher Channel because the entrance is less than 100 feet wide and the north side is encumbered by a rock. When we came through the next day after leaving Duncanby Landing, there were pine trees towering above the mast and on the tip of one tree, stoically guarding the entrance, was a majestic bald eagle. As we passed a waterfall cascading from the rock face of a high cliff off our starboard side, I immediately understood why they had set this area aside as a marine park. In this saltwater lake, the trees and grass grow right down to the waterline and mountains rise to 800 feet on all sides. The sharp, clear reflections in the mirror-still water play tricks with your mind, until you can hardly distinguish up from down. At sunset, later that night, I was reminded of a scene from the old movie with Henry Fonda and his daughter, Jane, *On Golden Pond*.

The next day we were headed for Shearwater, a small fishing resort along the Inside Passage where most cruising boats stop for fuel. Unaware that advance reservations were advisable, we waited several hours on the transient dock before a space with electric power opened up for us. This would prove to be one of the few stops along the way where we could socialize with other boats. A small flotilla of Nordhavn yachts arrived. I immediately introduced myself to the captains and crew of these boats. Before long, our new friends Christy and Bucky arrived and Sharon set about organizing dinner for ten at the only restaurant in town. We had a tremendous time with all these folks. The next day the weather was lousy, so we decided to hunker down and visit with these wonderful people a little longer. I was treated to an in-depth tour of one of the Nordhavns.

I was very excited to learn that Clark, from the sailing vessel Rikki Tiki Tavi, was anchored in a nearby cove. I'd first met Clark and his lovely wife, Nina, over the ham radio when we were in California's Channel Islands the preceding fall. What a coincidence, I thought, that he would only be nine miles away. I plotted the detour and the next morning we headed off for the short trip. Discovery Cove was a great find, just far enough off the main route of travel to be mostly deserted, yet close enough that we didn't mind the detour. The sharp granite faces on the cliffs above told the story of ancient glaciers grinding their way through these mountains. We had a fascinating time visiting with our friends and learning how they had built their 42-foot trimaran in their back yard over a span of 15 years. They also introduced us to their Hobie paddle, peddle and sail kayaks, which we both tried out. Sharon had wanted a kayak ever since I first introduced her to sailing, but with the disability in my left shoulder and Sharon's arthritis, neither one of us could paddle far enough to justify buying kayaks. After trying out the Hobie's peddles, however, that all changed. The very next day, I was on the satellite phone to a dealer in Port Townsend, Washington. We bought two of them over the phone right then and there and arranged to have them shipped directly to Juneau to coincide with our arrival a few weeks hence. While kayaking, Sharon and I had both noted the presence of huge, bright orange jellyfish. We were immediately warned that this variety, the Lions Mane, has a dangerous, debilitating sting and that they should be avoided at all costs.

The weather in Discovery Cove felt like a heat wave compared to what we'd experienced just a day before. I didn't want to leave and I grumbled as I took off my shorts, trading them for long underwear and jeans. On our way to Clothes Bay, near the First Nation's town of Klemtu, we had another great thrill of our adventurous voyage. I had learned soon after arriving in the Pacific Northwest to never set sail without being sure I had my camera in the cockpit with me. Today, that rule paid off. As we rounded a corner near the entrance to Finlayson Channel, Sharon sighted a humpback – no, two humpbacks – close aboard and heading right for the boat. I grabbed the camera and in a stroke of pure luck, managed to capture great shots of their tails as they sounded, one after the other.

We nearly missed one of the first breathtakingly spectacular experiences of our whole trip. As I researched potential anchorages and ports along the Inside Passage, Khutz Inlet off the Princess Royal Channel looked like a convenient spot to overnight.

219

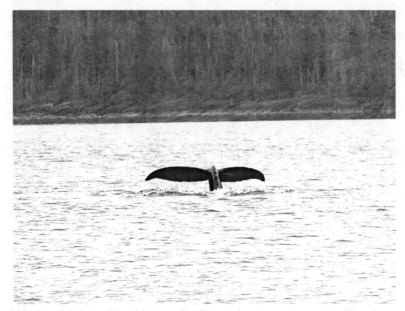

Whale-sightings like this one in Klemtu became commonplace in northern British Columbia and Alaska.

Together, the Princess Royal Channel and the Grenville Channel, into which it leads, are disparagingly referred to as the "Ditch." Both channels weave through deep slits cut into 125 miles of tree-covered hillside. While not particularly challenging, they do confront one with the need to carefully time passages with the incoming and outgoing tides, lest the currents slow progress to the point of making passage impractical. Douglass describes an anchorage about a mile inside Khutz Inlet, but discounts the benefit of proceeding the additional four miles to the head of this fiord. While we had seen lots of beautiful scenery prior to arriving here, this location thoroughly validated our decision to begin our life as cruising sailors in the Pacific Northwest. So steep were the sides of the fiord that satellite phone transmissions were impossible, but a few days later when I had Internet access, I gleefully circulated the spectacular pictures I'd captured here to our skeptical friends so they could see the scenic beauty we were enjoying.

This would be the first of many bear sightings. Fooled by our depth sounder, which was giving us false readings, apparently due

220

to the thermal layer caused by the cold water of the Khutz River colliding with the warmer sea water, we anchored in water that was far too deep on our first attempt. After I figured out the problem with the depth sounder, we managed to anchor very near the base of the incredible waterfall that cascaded down the lush green hillside, which was capped by stark white patches of snow, muted by encroaching banks of fog. No sooner had we affirmed that the anchor was securely set than we looked towards the waterfall and spotted our first grizzly. A huge, lumbering beast that had his nose nuzzled in the tall grass, disinterested in anything but the delicacies he hoped to find along the shoreline, now exposed by the receding tide. We watched, mesmerized, for what seemed like an hour.

Beyond our anchorage was a large meadow, framed by a backdrop of lush green mountains with much higher, snow-capped peaks looming farther behind. We couldn't wait to launch the dinghy. Frozen at first by the sight, we were too late to get close to the grizzly while he foraged on the shore, so we headed for the Khutz River, which we understood would be navigable in our small dinghy. As we entered the river there were steep mountains overgrown with dense brush on our port side and the broad meadow coming into clear view off our starboard quarter as we approached. Suddenly we spotted a black bear, followed closely by her two cavorting cubs, running, rolling and tumbling, until we lost site of their small bodies in the tall grass. So enthralled were we that we failed to notice the approach of a large male bear. The splash and ripple caused by this bear suddenly appearing from the tall grass and launching into the river heading directly towards us gave us both a heart-stopping moment. I slammed the outboard into reverse, but as I backed away it became clear that this bear only wanted to swim to the opposite shore. We'd been told that bears pay little mind to boats or people in the water. They don't perceive danger coming from the water so this bear simply didn't care that we were in his path.

Visiting with some other boaters who entered the anchorage later, we learned that the bears in this area are not to be trifled with, for this is a bear relocation area for animals that have created problems in prior encounters with humans. Enough said, we had no

221

desire from that point on to venture ashore. We hated to leave this place after only a day, but we had to keep moving. Sadly, we weren't planning on returning via the Ditch, so we might never see this unbelievable location again. I was thankful I owned a good camera and am a decent photographer, so the images were recorded digitally to be savored at a later time, when perhaps the memories dancing in the gray matter will begin to fade.

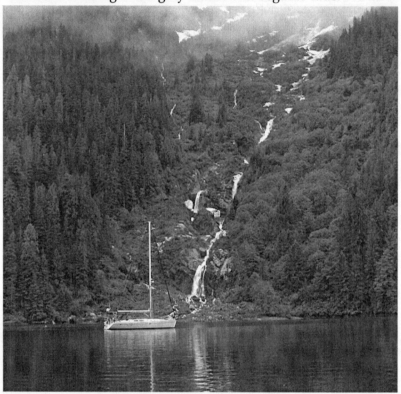

Anchored in Khutz Inlet, an isolated wonderland proves to be a chilly, but glorious, Shangri-La.

Looking for something to match our Khutz Inlet experience, I scoured the chart and cruising guide for a deserted anchorage to spend the next night. The cruising guide described what sounded like a remote spot, Hawk Bay on Fin Island, just a few miles off course from the point where the Princess Royal Channel meets the Glenville Channel. *En route* to Hawk Bay we passed nearby Hartley

222

Bay, a small First Nations settlement. On March 22, 2006, a British Columbia passenger ferry called *Queen of the North* sank in this area. It was a huge passenger ferry, capable of transporting 700 passengers and over 100 cars. Shortly after midnight, the ferry veered more than a mile off course. It struck a rock at Gil Island and sank. Fortunately, the crew of *Queen of the North* was able to evacuate almost all of the passengers before the boat sank. Most of the passengers were rescued from their lifeboats and taken to shore in the fishing boats of residents of Hartley Bay. Remarkably, 99 of the 101 passengers and crew survived the accident. This high survival rate is largely due to the extraordinary efforts of the residents of Hartley Bay. The following is a quote from the official investigation of the incident, "Essentially, the system failed that night. Sound watch-keeping practices were not followed and the bridge watch lacked a third certified person." The duty crew was uncooperative during the official investigations. Nobody is officially talking about it, but rumors abound in Hartley Bay that the two officers on duty, one male, the other female, were not at their posts and perhaps lust had overcome duty that fateful night.

We were in for a surprise when we arrived at Hawk Bay, for it was anything but the deserted cove described in the cruising guide. Right in front of us, looming large and occupying the entire head of the cove, was a hotel. That's right, a hotel – lights blazing, guests buzzing and noises emanating – in the middle of what we'd assumed would be an idyllic, secluded location. Nothing to be done for it, we dropped the anchor and watched as the fishing boats darted to and fro and the occasional sea plane landed within 50 feet of our bow, depositing hopeful anglers and picking up the less fortunate, those heading back to home and office. Thinking we should make the best of it, I hailed one of the passing boats and hitched a ride to this floating hotel, hoping to make dinner reservations and treat Sharon to a night out of the galley. I soon found the proprietor, who was very friendly and explained that each year they towed this "hotel" from Nanaimo to this small bay to operate as a fishing lodge, but who nevertheless firmly advised me that dinner was only for the guests and Sharon and I would not be welcome. "Humph," I thought, as I hoped he'd at least be good enough to provide a return trip out to our boat.

I'd already formed a better opinion of the Ditch than most, having experienced Khutz Inlet, so I was optimistic as we set forth for Baker Inlet. It sounded scenic from the descriptions I'd read, but I was at once both fearful and curious about the passage through Watts Narrows that would be required to enter the inlet. I took one look at the narrow, winding, blind channel, which seemed to have way too much current for slack tide and thought to myself, "Are you kidding?" With trees overhanging this already constricted channel, I thought we'd surely snag a branch in our rig or that the tide tables were wrong and we'd be dashed on one of the threatening rocks lining the shore as we ventured into this labyrinth. After issuing a prudent Securité call over the VHF radio to announce that we were entering the blind channel, we twisted and turned and edged our way through. At times we had less than ten feet between ourselves and the rocky shore. We soon spied the safety of Baker

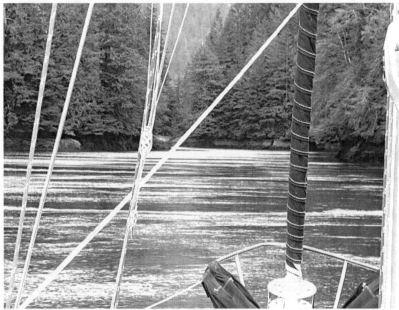

Navigating through twisting, blind Watts Narrows had me clinging to the sailing instructions like a life raft.

Inlet, if only we could negotiate the last turn. The effort to challenge the narrows did not disappoint us, for Baker Inlet was majestic in its own right. The surrounding mountains were punctuated with ribbons of waterfalls appearing in every possible crevice and crack. We enjoyed our evening there and even had cocktails aboard a large powerboat that anchored nearby an hour or two after our arrival. I was left wondering what manner of current he'd encountered in Watts Narrows, since they clearly didn't pass at slack tide. My query was met with an artful dodge from the captain and a groan from his wife that said it all.

I didn't care for our next stop at all. Prince Rupert is the only significant town on the north coast of British Columbia and its reputation of being an unfriendly place for cruisers is legendary. Upon our arrival, we discovered we were out of luck and couldn't find space at the yacht club, the only decent moorage that welcomed pleasure boats. A radio call for advice only resulted in an unfriendly and less-than-helpful response that we should put in at the public float. The only public floats we'd seen were already packed with gnarly fishing boats rafted three deep, a rather uninviting prospect with our shiny new white hull. I finally found a dock with room for us, but we'd no sooner tied up than a nearby fisherman told us it was the private dock of the local cannery. Since it was Sunday, he didn't think that would be a problem, so with no power or water and enduring the numerous wakes of ships, and even sea planes, passing by up and down the channel, we suffered through an uncomfortable night worrying about what the cannery owners might say in the morning.

Rather than wait around to find out, since the place was singularly unpleasant, we decided to just push on. This was the day we would enter Alaska and we were brimming with excitement and anticipation. The plan was to top off the fuel tanks and get an early start, so at 7:00 a.m. sharp we pulled up to the fuel dock. When another waiting boat told us they didn't open until 7:30 a.m. and that was only if the attendant showed up for work on time, I made a quick fuel calculation and decided we should push on. The tide was with us, but we needed to move on quickly, so at near full throttle we started the last leg to Alaska. Every vessel entering

225

Alaska has to go to Ketchikan to clear customs, but there is an exception for slower-moving boats that can't make the 90-mile trip in one day. It is possible to obtain clearance to anchor in Foggy Bay, the first possible place to stop when entering Alaska from Canada. That was our plan, but fighting the tide we were starting to burn our dwindling fuel at an alarming rate. Rather than risk running out with the small detour and the possibility of needing fuel to power the generator overnight, we decided to push on.

An hour from the international border we anxiously started counting down the minutes. We were within striking distance of our goal. Alaska was dead ahead. I wanted to take a picture of the chartplotter display as we entered Alaska and I thought I'd get a better shot of the repeated display on the large plasma television below decks than I would on the smaller display in the cockpit. I left Sharon at the helm as we approached the imaginary point that marked the boundary and went below to set up for the shot. We were a split second from the border and I'd started focusing the camera when the boat lurched into a radical turn to port. Anxious for an explanation, I raced up the companionway stairs and all but launched myself into the cockpit. When I arrived, Sharon nervously explained that a humpback whale had surfaced directly in front of the boat and she had no other alternative but to make an emergency course change or run down the unsuspecting whale. I wasn't convinced. Once back on course I quickly darted below to catch my picture at the moment of arrival.

Jubilant at defying the odds and surviving to fulfill a lifelong dream of sailing to Alaska, we had a celebration in the cockpit. Sharon took the American flag out of its holder on the stern rail and triumphantly waved it about as we danced to the strains of Neil Diamond's *"Coming to America."*

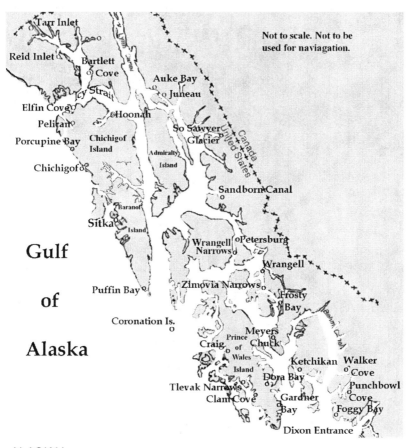

Not to scale. Not to be
used for naviagation.

Tarr Inlet

Reid Inlet

Bartlett
Cove

Auke Bay

Juneau

Icy Strait

Elfin Cove

Pelican

Hoonah

So Sawyer
Glacier

Porcupine Bay

Chichigof
Island

Chichigof

Admiralty

Island

Canada
United States

Chichigof

Baranof

Sandborn Canal

Sitka

Island

Gulf

Wrangell
Narrows

Petersburg

Wrangell

Puffin Bay

of

Zimovia Narrows

Frosty
Bay

Coronation Is.

Alaska

Meyers
Chuck

Craig

Prince

of

Wales

Island

Ketchikan

Walker
Cove

Dora Bay

Punchbowl
Cove

Tlevak Narrows

Clam Cove

Gardner
Bay

Foggy Bay

Dixon Entrance

ALASKA!

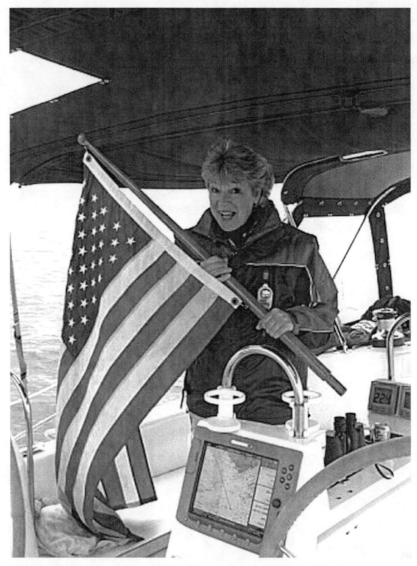

Sharon's a Yankee Doodle Dandy, once we arrive in Alaskan waters.

Chapter 10
"Just Man Up"

As we caught our first glimpse of Alaska I was immediately reminded of a comment our friend Terri had made shortly before we left San Francisco, "Everything in Alaska is big!" What I saw as we crossed Dixon Entrance was majestic. There was a marked difference as towering mountains, burdened by perennial fields of snow, came into view, and the steely blue water faded to an opaque gray, deep and forbidding.

Ketchikan was only a few hours ahead now that we'd made the decision to bypass Foggy Bay. I nervously eyed the fuel gauges and anxiously counted down the minutes until the next tide change. I was relying on the boost we'd get from the current to reduce our fuel consumption sufficiently to get us to Ketchikan before running dry. Maybe I'd been too compulsive leaving Prince Rupert without topping off the tanks. At this moment I was regretting selling all the jerry jugs, thinking it would have been a good idea to have had a five-gallon reserve stashed away somewhere.

I tried not to dwell on this concern for long, because I was enthralled by the scenery that filled the eye and touched every sense. There had been no wind all day and as a result the seas across Dixon Entrance had been relatively flat. As we approached Revillagigedo Channel leading to Ketchikan, a respectable breeze began to build, but not enough to supplant the engine. We wanted to get there as fast as possible, not to mention the U.S. Customs office closes at 5:00 p.m. We didn't want to pay overtime charges for a late arrival. But I was relieved because at least we could sail into port if fuel became critical.

Ketchikan's harbor department assigns arriving vessels to one of three available marinas. Everything is on a first-come, first-served basis, so we were hoping we'd be assigned to Thomas Basin. Of the three, this is the most desirable location. While it's adjacent to the cruise ship docks, it is also in the heart of town close to most of the services and entertainment. Luck was with us. We were even more thrilled when our friends from the Nordhavn group, and Bucky aboard his trawler, were all waiting for us and even helped us dock. They had heard of our arrival when we called the harbormaster on our VHF radio. What a pleasant surprise. We hadn't seen any of them for over a week. Since their powerboats were all slightly faster than *Last Resort*, we didn't know if we'd catch up with them again or not, having left them when we detoured to Discovery Cove. We immediately organized a dinner on the town for the next night and set about cleaning up the boat and getting organized.

Now that we were in Alaska, I thought we could slow down the pace. I was determined to amass all the fishing gear I'd need to catch crabs and salmon. After the dockmaster took down all the vital information and we'd paid for our slip, we both sat down to relax and catch our breath. We planned to spend a week in Ketchikan. We needed rest, I had to retrieve our latest batch of mail from Scottsdale and there were any number of ship's matters calling for my attention. I also wanted to take advantage of the cell phone service to access the Internet and update my website. I hadn't changed it since we arrived in Port Angeles and there was so much information and hundreds of pictures to Photoshop and upload. I didn't know if there would be sufficient space to tell the whole story.

We enjoyed lovely weather the first few days in Ketchikan. I was able to effectively use my scooter as I ran all over town collecting things we'd need for the summer in Alaska. I tried to get television reception using satellite settings I'd obtained directly from SeaTel before leaving the continental United States, but hard as I tried, Dish Network's Alaska satellite would not come into line-of-sight from our location. After I got my fishing license, I sat down to read and absorb the regulations. I was distracted by the governor's picture on the back cover. I commented to Sharon, as I showed her the picture, what an attractive woman I thought Governor Sarah Palin was. Without television, I had no idea of the fire storm that would surround Sarah Palin in the weeks and months to come and the fun we'd all have at her expense, especially Democrats and Tina Fey from *Saturday Night Live*, who did a masterful job of parodying

Palin after Senator John McCain unexpectedly and dramatically picked her as his running mate.

In addition to shopping and attending to ship's business, we also made the rounds of all the tourist sights. After a few days, our friends had all moved on and we had little else to do. We wandered up Creek Street, an entire city block or two, constructed completely on a boardwalk straddling the creek that ran through town. We decided to take a tour of Dolly's House, an infamous brothel that was closed in the Fifties under pressure from the U. S. Coast Guard. I made a startling and somewhat nostalgic discovery as we toured the dining room. For most of his career, my late father had worked for Gladding McBean, the manufacturers of Franciscan Ware china. The top of their line was the Rose pattern, which we used in our own home when I was a kid. Dolly obviously had good taste, because the table boasted a setting for eight of this fine china. My father would have found some irony in this, I'm sure.

We'd suggested to our friends that before they left all of us should go to the Great Alaskan Lumberjack show, even though it exists primarily for the cruise ship passengers. They had scoffed at the idea, but we decided to attend the show anyway, after they all left town. We had a great time, and while it was pretty hokey, the athletes were actually very impressive. One of the athletes was third in the world at the pole climb. During the competition, he was up and down a 50-foot pole before his competitor could even make it halfway up his own pole.

While most of the other boats were already continuing north in the direction of Wrangell, Petersburg and Juneau, we had been reading about the Misty Fiords National Monument and decided we'd take a long detour, even backtrack a little to get there. Our first stop was Punchbowl Cove, one of several inlets. After anchoring, we took a long dinghy ride and photographed what seemed like hundreds of waterfalls that emptied into this bay along every few yards of the meandering, sheer shoreline.

Meanwhile, my computer was continuing to crash every time we had a power glitch. This night I lost all the entries in the ship's log that I'd made since the last back-up I'd done to my spare hard drive while in Port Hardy. Frustrated beyond endurance, I restored

231

the hard drive to that point, and as I racked my brain to recreate the log, I vowed to replace Vista with Windows XP at my earliest opportunity. It was too bad. I liked Vista, but it was too unstable for the demanding ship-board environment and marine software programs.

The next day we headed deeper into the fiords, our destination being Walker Cove, where we'd read there was another mooring buoy. Somebody needed to pinch me to make me believe we were really sailing our own boat into this breathtaking fiord. I'd never seen anything like it and briefly lost myself in daydreams. I had no idea that Alaska had fiords rivaling those of Scandinavia, which I'd first studied in junior high school. We'd been sailing downwind and making good time for the last 20 miles and we were still sailing as we reached the first cove, where we discovered the only U.S. Forest Service mooring buoy in all of Walker Cove was occupied. Not one to be dissuaded, I ventured farther into the fiord. Seven miles deep we were treated to the vista of another glacial valley ending in a grassy marsh, much of which was submerged at high tide. Anchoring in the deep water was difficult, but after two tries we were successful and anchored in 120 feet, our deepest anchorage ever.

Once we were set I couldn't wait to deploy our new crab and prawn pots. This was our first try and we did it without too much trouble, although once while the heavy leaded line was paying out with the prawn pot, I wrapped my ankle and had to react quickly lest I be pulled off the dinghy by the combined weight and momentum of the rapidly sinking pot and line. I didn't think we'd set the prawn pot in deep enough water, as it was only in about 120 feet. Three or four hundred feet would have been a lot better. I had higher hopes for the crab pot.

Once back on board, I settled down to work on email, but in the depths of this superior fiord I couldn't get the single sideband radio or the satellite phone to work. We were totally isolated. Before I could fret about it for long, Sharon stuck her head through the companionway and announced that there was a mother grizzly with two cubs in the marsh ashore. Now that was something to behold. We watched them for almost two hours, but since we were both really exhausted, we went to bed early. By now, darkness was falling later and later, a dramatic change caused by the normal lengthening of summer days, which was exaggerated by our northward progress of close to 50 miles a day.

In the morning, I hurriedly dressed warmly to go out and retrieve the pots. After hauling in the prawn pot I was disappointed, but not altogether surprised, when it came up empty. Expecting the same, I didn't pay a lot of attention when I pulled in the crab pot. I was pretty startled when I discovered a large crab cowering inside. Shaking from excitement, I set about cleaning it with only the benefit of some hastily delivered instructions the kid in the sporting goods store in Ketchikan had given me when I bought the equipment. At this instant I wished I'd paid closer attention.

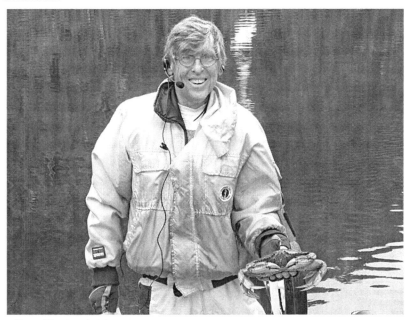

Deadliest catch!

Sharon teased me to no end about this lone crab and later she actually put her mocking commentary in writing in an email to Terri and Kimi:

> You should have seen us deploying these traps for the

first time. We bumbled around like first-graders with a chemistry set. We spent the good part of an evening dropping the two pots and the next morning I sent forth our great white hunter to collect the proceeds. He pulled up the prawn pot; no dough. He pulled up the crab pot, and lo and behold, one (1) crab! He nearly jumped out of the dinghy in surprise. Later he quipped, "It was like the Deadliest Catch!"

Crab pot — $100
Shrimp pot — $120
Other junk — $200
The joy in finally catching a crab? Priceless

The next few days were a whirlwind. When we left Walker Cove we elected to continue all the way through the Behm Canal, which rejoins Clarence Strait just 10 miles north of Ketchikan, bringing us full circle. We couldn't help but notice the chalky green, almost tropical, color of the water as we sailed deeper into Misty Fiords. We'd read about the prevalence of glacial silt in Alaskan waters, but seeing it first-hand I began to grow concerned about our ability to make water. Places to fill the water tanks would be few and far between as we got farther north, so it would be important to top them off whenever possible and to use the watermaker carefully, lest we ruin the filters.

We stopped that night in Helm Bay, after a very long day's sail, where we were able to tie up to an Alaska State Float. There was nothing much to see there, so we left with the tide early the next morning headed for Meyers Chuck. The waters in Clarence Strait looked pretty clear so I decided to make water. I made a big mistake. I'd closed all the valves the last time we'd finished making water and forgot to open one so the water could feed into an empty tank. By the time I realized my error it was too late. The fine tubing that carried the product water from the watermaker to the manifold where it was distributed to an appropriate tank had already ruptured and water was spewing throughout the bilge. I also damaged the compression fittings on each end of that 10-foot long tube and they were leaking as well. Thoroughly annoyed with myself, I

234

asked Sharon to drive and I buried my head in the bilge to repair the damages. Totally preoccupied, I failed to notice that the winds outside had built to 25-to-30 knots. After I managed to jury-rig a temporary repair and stop the leaks, I went upstairs and was stunned to see what Sharon had been dealing with. There were angry whitecaps everywhere and Sharon had to hand-steer because the gusting winds on the over-sheeted headsail were over-powering the autopilot. I was proud of her for dealing with these conditions on her own. Sharon was showing signs of completing her personal "inside passage" that she'd so passionately written about earlier.

When we finally arrived, we found Meyers Chuck to be an eclectic little berg. The town was built around a small cove, while the post office and some other essential services had been built on a small island that sheltered the cove from wind-swept Clarence Strait. Every house had a small dock and they must have all bought their bright red skiffs from the same dealer. Poking around, we came upon a small art gallery that only opened by appointment. Someone with a good sense of humor had constructed a huge spider web by stretching string from tree to tree. It must have measured 20 feet-by-20 feet, complete with a sculpted iron spider. I chuckled as I photographed this local art and wondered about the nature of these Alaskans that would lead them to tiny little bergs so totally isolated from the main stream of society. I managed to reach the watermaker dealer before we left Meyers Chuck and placed an order for parts to replace my temporary repairs.

Our next stop as we pushed on was Frosty Bay. There was a bear-viewing station another 25 miles farther ahead. It was out of the way, so we elected to anchor overnight in Frosty Bay and push on to Wrangell the next day. Since it looked to be a likely spot, I decided to drag out the new halibut gear I'd purchased and have a go at it. Sharon apparently hadn't quite gotten over the mocking mood she'd been in when we caught the crab at Walker Cove, because that night she wrote another email to Terri:

> Last night Dick decided he would catch a halibut. eu,niyndfkljwehfnv [Excuse me, I was still laughing.] "I'm jigging," he explains. He is jerking his fishing pole up and

235

down like a carousel pony. "It's when you lure the halibut into thinking there's a smaller fish in trouble that will be easy prey." He has bathed his colorful lure with very aptly-named Butt Juice. The lure's yellow and white streamers flutter very attractively. As we wait, he tries different techniques. First there is the straight up and down jig. This is akin to the missionary position in jigging and it is not exciting to watch or participate in, apparently. So he enhances his repertoire to include exotic moves like figure eights, before introducing increasingly higher levels of difficulty. "That's good," I encourage him. "That must look like final death throes down there. I'm sure it's like Madame Butterfly."

Did I happen to mention that I've been appointed to the position of Gaffer? The Gaffer gets to take this pole with a steel hook on the end, poke it into the halibut's gill whenever Dick pulls it out of the water and hold the approximately 100-pound fish thusly, until Dick manages to do something about it. (What that something was has yet to be explained or probably even thought through, exactly.) Fortunately, halibut did not apparently find our Butt Juice stimulating enough. I ate chicken last night."

Much to my chagrin, I learned that Terri was sharing this email with everyone she knew in San Francisco. I was sure they were all having a good laugh at my expense.

The next day we headed to Wrangell. From Ketchikan there are a couple of different routes that can be followed to reach Wrangell, but by committing to Frosty Bay, I'd already selected the more difficult route through Zimovia Strait. The sailing instructions caution that this route, especially the critical part of the passage through the Zimovia Narrows, requires careful navigation. I thought it would be good practice for Wrangell Narrows, the infamous dredged canal that lay beyond the town of Wrangell itself. We'd left Frosty Bay in a flurry earlier that morning when Sharon reported that the satellite phone wasn't getting a signal for one of her scheduled conference calls. She also reported seeing an orange float, exactly like the one we'd deployed when we set the crab pot the night before, bobbing lose as it was swept away by the current. I felt pressure to hurry, so quickly weighing anchor, we motored over to where we'd left the crab pot. It was there, but only yielded one starfish. We barely got it aboard and stowed in time for Sharon to make her conference call. Communications were getting more and more challenging. Our Verizon Aircards were prohibitively expensive in Canada, so we didn't use them at all while we were there. We'd reactivated them in Ketchikan, but cell service was all but non-existent.

Running the Zimovia Narrows *en route* to Wrangell was a new challenge, unlike anything I'd ever encountered before, with some of the buoys actually requiring us to back-track to round them. Bodega Bay came to mind as I wound around this complex maze of buoys. A navigation error here could have had dire consequences, given the rate of flow of the currents in the narrows. After we cleared the narrows we made very good time to Wrangell, where we arrived early that afternoon.

We re-provisioned in Wrangell, where I also bought a new fishing reel and rented a movie, since we were unsuccessful in connecting to the Dish Network satellite that provides coverage to Alaska. The world was going on, but we were oblivious to it all. I missed a lot of the election news, but I'd long ago lost my passion for 24/7 cable news. I partially blamed the stress that resulted from watching so much of it as another possible reason I'd been stricken with cancer.

Wrangell Narrows can best be described as a piloting challenge. There are over 60 numbered navigational aids, including five sets of range markers, along this 21-mile, narrow channel. Constant vigilance is required so as not to miss any of the marks, since wandering outside the dredged channel in some spots would result in immediate grounding. It turns out we were lucky and didn't meet any oncoming tugs with log booms or ferry boats in narrow areas that would have made passing a dangerous challenge. Once safely in Petersburg, the XO and I found it very satisfying to include our passage through Wrangell Narrows among our cruising accomplishments.

Petersburg looked like a cute town, but we never saw it. We hunkered down inside our cozy boat all day and night, sheltering from the pouring rain which was flying horizontally in the ferocious winds that howled through our rigging. We were sorry to leave in the morning without ever going into town, but there simply didn't seem to be enough there to warrant staying another day. The promise of seeing our first glaciers was only a half-day's sail ahead and that lured us more than any attraction the town might hold.

With good wind and favorable current, we made it to our next stop, Sandborn Canal, in record time. On the way we saw our first glacier, Leconte Glacier, albeit from a distance, but it was spectacular and we were awed to see a glacier first hand. We also saw 10 humpback whales during this trip, two that breached, the first time we'd seen that since arriving in Alaska. It was a day of discovery. The cruising guide said we might encounter icebergs from here on, but we didn't see any that day. Sandborn Canal is deep inside Houghton Bay, but looked nice enough to warrant the 10 miles we'd gone out of our way to get there and back. It was a good anchorage and since it was full of crab pots, we thought we'd give it a try too. We spent a quiet night. The crab pot came up empty the next morning. The place was either fished out or we'd picked a bad spot, trying too hard to stay well clear of all the other pots that were already there. We'd later come to learn something else about Sandborn Canal that we wouldn't soon forget.

The next day would prove to be very exciting. It would take us to Tracy Arm, site of South Sawyer Glacier, the first glacier we would have a chance to see up close, if only we could successfully negotiate our way through the pack ice that reportedly often clogs the 21-mile fiord leading to the glacier. I noticed on the way there that the knotmeter wasn't working and made a mental note to pull the sending unit and find out what was blocking it when we were safely anchored that night. As we approached Tracy Arm, I saw something off in the distance that looked like a large power boat. After awhile, I began to notice that it wasn't moving. It was only after I got closer and took a look through the binoculars that I discovered I was actually looking at my first iceberg.

238

We saw a small cruise ship leaving Tracy Arm, and by picking up his call sign from the AIS display, I was able to radio him to inquire about ice conditions at the glaciers. We were told that we might be able to get up to South Sawyer glacier, but we'd have to be careful because the ice was pretty thick. There is a shallow bar with a narrow opening that must be crossed to enter and depart Tracy Arm. The path of entry is so critical that vessel-operated range lights and day beacons have been installed to keep boats from straying out of the channel. The buoys are unreliable because icebergs frequently drag them off station, an accident waiting to happen for the unsuspecting mariner. We navigated carefully and as we entered we were in awe of what we saw. I remember writing in the log book that it was like nothing I'd ever seen or could really imagine. I suspect a lot of people have seen this area, or if not, Glacier Bay, but seeing it from the relative safety of a cruise ship is nothing like encountering icebergs as big as houses, with dozens of much smaller ones that could slash our vulnerable fiberglass hull as easily as the Titanic. As a friend of mine had said earlier, when

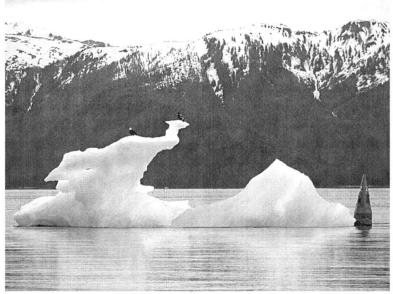

Icebergs leaving Tracy Arm with the ebbing tide frequently tow this navigation buoy off-station.

contemplating sailing a fiberglass boat through this minefield, "Put the emphasis on *glass!*"

Icebergs take on a beautiful blue color because the ice is so compressed that all of the air has literally been squeezed out of them. It is said that by the time an iceberg calves from a glacier, the ice is over 10,000 years old. Try this in your 12-year old single malt scotch! Because it was late and we'd already sailed 40 miles, we decided to venture a short distance up the fiord just to get a feel for it. We planned to return early the next morning, when the tide would be more favorable and we'd be refreshed and ready for our attempt to reach the base of South Sawyer Glacier.

As if we didn't have enough to worry about with uncharted rocks, raging, turbulent currents, williwaws (a type of katabatic wind that results from the descent of cold, dense air from the snow and ice fields of the coastal mountains, accelerated by the force of gravity), deadhead logs, violent storms, crab pots, big seas, life-threatening mechanical failures, and cruise ships in narrow channels, we could now add "bergy bits" to our list. Bergy bits are small fragments of larger icebergs that can lurk at or below the surface. Cruise ships exacerbate the problem of bergy bits because they churn up larger pieces, breaking them into smaller ones. Bergy bits may sound cute, but they are harder to see than large icebergs and can easily render a small propeller useless. Make no mistake about it, this was serious sailing. The water temperature was near freezing and even with a life jacket, hypothermia could set in almost immediately and life expectancy would be less than 15 minutes should one of us fall overboard. Loss of propulsion or damage to our rudder would have left us at the mercy of the endless parade of marching icebergs. Large icebergs can topple over with enough force to crush our vulnerable boat, or we could drift or be driven helplessly into the sheer rock cliffs that lined the narrow channel. We were beyond radio range or any chance of summoning help if we had a problem. We were on our own and great care had to be taken.

We only made it eight miles into the fiord that afternoon, and since the sun was already behind the surrounding peaks, it seemed prudent to head back to William Cove, an anchorage we'd spotted on the way in, for the night. Once there, we found another boat occupying the small anchorage, but with the help of a stern line led ashore in the dinghy and tied off to a tree, we were secure for the night.

When I noted that the knotmeter wasn't working earlier in the day, I assumed it had some growth on it and that when we headed out into Stephens Passage, with 20-knot winds on the nose and three-to-four foot seas, it would shake lose. Well, it didn't. So now that we were anchored, I pulled the knotmeter and was stunned to find a bunch of little bugs growing and living in the paddle wheel. They looked like what I call pill bugs and Sharon calls roly-poly bugs – those little gray bugs you find in the garden that roll up in a ball when you disturb them. Apparently there is a waterborne variety unique to Alaska. They look like something from prehistoric times. I cleaned them out and replaced the knotmeter, but suddenly a cold sweat came over me and I stopped in my tracks. What about the other thru-hulls? The first place I went was to the sea strainer on the engine, and sure enough, it had so many of those things clogging it that I was surprised the engine wasn't overheating. How was I going to get rid of these things? They appeared to be multiplying rapidly, based on the number of really tiny, newborn looking specimens. This was serious. If the smaller ones got through the strainer and started multiplying in the cooling system or the heat exchanger, our engine would be disabled and we'd be in serious danger. I hadn't even looked at the generator yet, and what about the bathroom heads, which were drawing salt water too. I tried drowning the engine cooling system sea strainer with Clorox. I couldn't believe it. These things weren't bothered by it at all. They just swam around like it was business as usual.

This was becoming a scene from a bad horror movie. Bill Alland could have made a fortune turning this story into a script for one of his B-rated science fiction movies. I resorted to the ham radio. We didn't have a safety net 'for nothing' and surely someone would know the answer. The Alaska Bush Net was in progress when I tuned in, so I waited for the appropriate break in the net's business to break in. The description of my plight brought all other network business to an immediate halt. But sadly, nobody had heard of this issue before. Unlike the morning net, which is primarily for sailors and marine interests, the Alaska Bush Net didn't have many sailors and maybe only a fisherman or two. They tried to be helpful, but I was wasting precious time and politely begged off to find another solution.

I captured a few of these little beasts and tested some wasp and hornet spray to see if it would kill them. It said on the can that this stuff is harmful to fish and marine life. "Fantastic, bring it on," I thought. It looked like I was in luck, because they died instantly, turning a milky white color in the process. All the deader I thought. I sprayed almost a cup-full in the seawater strainer, and after seeing that the bugs were dead, thoroughly removed the bug spray before running the engine for a few seconds. I prayed they hadn't reached the engine, because even a dead one would clog the narrow tubing of the heat exchanger. Who knew how long the skeletal remains of these little creatures would take to decay, even in the near-boiling hot exhaust water produced by the engine? I planned to let it sit overnight and treat it again before running the engine again in the morning. That done I checked the generator, but since I hadn't run it in Sandborn Canal, where we undoubtedly picked up this infestation, it appeared to be clear. Oh no, I thought, had I dropped any of them into the bilge when I pulled the sending unit on the knotmeter and had started knocking them off without, at first, thinking about the possible consequences? I didn't want to take any chances, so notwithstanding the strong smell, I sprayed the bilge down thoroughly with the poison to be sure I'd kill any that remained. We were sure we'd eradicated the infestation. When it was all over, Sharon and I fell into a breathless, giddy laughing fit, comparing ourselves to Captain Kirk on the Starship Enterprise in the episode, "The Trouble with Tribbles."

In the morning, we left the anchorage very early to catch the flood tide as we headed up the fiord, so by 8:00 a.m. we were way too deep in the steep canyons to contact the Great Northern Boater's Net. I was sure they'd heard our story by now and would be wondering our fate. Nothing to be done for it, we had a much bigger adventure dead ahead of us. As we ventured farther and farther, the canyon walls closed in and the icebergs were growing larger and getting closer together, too. The depth for most of the trip was beyond the range of our depth sounder, but at one point it suddenly shot up to 15 feet, measured from the bottom of our eight foot keel. Before I could react it went off the scale again. I wondered what happened and when I looked back, thinking I'd see debris or something in the water, I was stunned to see a pod of Orcas surface close astern. They had passed directly under the boat. Good thing they didn't have any reason to want to stave our hull. It was eerie, especially watching those dorsal fins that really resembled a periscope when viewed from directly in front or from behind. I have to admit my stress level was rising as we neared the ice that I knew was waiting around any corner now.

We traveled 15 miles before we encountered ice too thick to allow our unimpeded passage. When we were about four miles from South Sawyer Glacier the ice started getting really thick. I positioned Sharon on the bow with a headset to alert me to any icebergs or bergy bits I might not see and a boat hook to fend them off in an emergency, but it was freezing cold outside by now, so she didn't last long up there exposed to the oncoming wind. We slowed to a crawl and threaded our way through as best we could. When the prop hit a bergy bit it was time to stop. I decided to launch the dinghy and see if I could get farther up. I was scared, but I didn't want to miss the opportunity. I dressed in as many layers of warm clothes as I could, and praying Sharon wouldn't have any problems, I set out. I was able to make really good time in the dinghy by maneuvering around all the bergy bits that littered the path. When I was within a mile of the glacier I got my first view. My breathing must have stopped for a full minute as I gazed in awe at South Sawyer Glacier. It was huge and it had the appearance of a mile-high tidal wave – like the ones you see in those asteroid-hits-Earth movies – just waiting to come crashing down the fiord, swamping me, my dinghy, and poor Sharon waiting helplessly three miles downstream. I kept going for about another half-mile, but by now, I was dangerously close to icebergs as big as buses that dwarfed my tiny dinghy, and I was starting to hit small pieces of ice. My mind was setting off discordant warning bells and I didn't relish rowing three miles to get back to the mother ship in this freezing cold if my prop should be damaged. Even wearing big ski gloves layered over a pair of tight-fitting latex gloves, my hands were frozen. It was time to go back. After taking as many pictures as I could in the few moments my hands could endure after taking off the big outer gloves to manipulate the camera, I turned around and covered the three miles back to Sharon pretty quickly.

She was fine, but I was too chilled to pull the dingy up on the davits immediately, so I asked her if she'd keep watch a little longer while I thawed out below and had some lunch. She'd discovered that if she turned off the engine, she would drift at the same rate as the ice, reducing the chance of colliding with an iceberg. She'd been able to go below to eat lunch herself, so she was warmed and fed. After I warmed up, we stowed the dinghy and motored until we cleared the worst of the ice. The wind had really picked up and it was getting warmer as we put distance between ourselves and the glacier. We decided to raise the sails and proceed without the motor, enjoying the silence of this stark, ice-filled no-man's land. It was an odd feeling to glide silently by the beautiful, blue hulking icebergs.

We were originally planning to stay another night in Tracy Arm, but we'd gotten word that our new Hobie kayaks were going to arrive in Juneau in two days, so we decided to push on and stop for the night when we were closer to Juneau. I believe that the solo dinghy trip to Sawyer Glacier is one of the most dangerous and exhilarating things I've ever done. I'd survived cancer and I was living life to its fullest. I couldn't imagine a more exciting adventure.

We found a little place called Taku Harbor that had a comfortable public float where we tied up and spent a restful night. Without any worries about runaway icebergs, a dragging anchor or little bugs taking over the engine, I fell asleep quickly and slept like a baby. When we awoke it was raining, but it was time to go. We were only 35 miles from Auke Bay, so if we hurried, we had a chance of getting our kayaks that very day. Sailboats our size can't actually moor in Juneau. The pleasure boat marina can only be accessed by passing under a 50-foot bridge and our 65-foot mast obviously can't clear it, even at extreme low tide, or at least I wouldn't chance it or run the risk of getting hopelessly trapped. Auke Bay is where most of the pleasure boats and all the sailboats visiting the Juneau-area end up. This marina has no permanent berths and imposes a 10-day time limit before you are required to leave. It is a huge marina with almost 8,000 linear feet of dock space. I don't know how many boats it can hold, but it's a bunch.

We arrived in Auke Bay at 12:30 p.m. The reality just hadn't sunk in yet. We had now logged over 2600 nautical miles (the equivalent of over 3100 statute miles, had we driven the same distance in a car) since leaving Mexico. It seemed like an incredible feat to us, but the impact of it all was lost with the tasks at hand and the sheer enormity of our surroundings. We had an unobstructed view of nearby Mendenhall Glacier right from the cockpit. We had things to do and no time to waste. Once the lines were tied securely and we'd hooked up the shore power, I set off to check in with the marina office, but before I left, I placed a call to Ben, the fellow who was going to help us with our kayaks. Our new friend Stephanie, from the Half Moon Bay Yacht Club, had a friend whose sister lived in Juneau with her husband, Ben. He had a truck and was gracious enough to agree to take us to the warehouse to pick up our kayaks. He couldn't break away from the office until 3:00 p.m., but as long as we got there by 4:00 p.m., we were told we'd be able to retrieve the kayaks, which fortuitously arrived the same day.

As I walked down the dock, one of the boats I passed had a familiar look. It didn't register immediately because it didn't have the traditional blue and silver stripes that distinguish recent-vintage Catalina yachts. I walked about 20 feet past this boat when the synapses connected. I stopped dead in my tracks, wheeled around and started knocking on the hull. A burly, bearded figure emerged and before I even asked, I knew I was looking at Lou. There were only two Catalina 470s that I'm aware of that have ever sailed in Alaskan waters. Ours was one and *Seventh Heaven*, owned by Lou and Mary, the other. Lou and I had corresponded for over a year through the C470 Association's message board, and while we were aware of each other's plans to sail to Alaska, we'd made no arrangements to rendezvous. And yet here we were, just two slips apart. They had only arrived about an hour ahead of us. The coincidence was remarkable. I couldn't linger at that moment because I was obligated to check in with the marina office and we had to eat before Ben arrived to pick us up, but we made plans to get together during the evening.

Ben was a great guy. Not only did he drive us to the warehouse and back with our kayaks loaded on his truck, he also stayed around and helped us unpack, assemble and launch them. Ben worked for the local maritime union and was very popular with the marina staff, so while we peddled and paddled the new kayaks from the launch ramp back to the boat, he visited with friends in the office before coming down to the boat for a drink and snacks. He had other obligations and couldn't stay for dinner. His wife was out of town, but we hoped we might see them when she returned and before we left Auke Bay. We would have, too, except the cell service was unreliable and we missed a phone call and the message they left extending an invitation to an Independence Day party at their house. This was upsetting, but there was little we could do about it. The date was July 1. We had arrived five days ahead of Stephen and Katie's scheduled flight. We had plenty of time to regroup, explore Juneau and get some much needed rest. We'd also have a chance to familiarize ourselves with the new kayaks in the relative safety of the marina before we put them to a real test in Glacier Bay.

We enjoyed a relaxing week in Auke Bay, shopping, sightseeing and visiting with our new friends Lou and Mary, cleaning and planning in between. I also managed to find a store that had a solution to my computer problems. They didn't think my Hewlett Packard computer that came with Vista installed would be compatible with Windows XP without a lot of work to find the appropriate drivers, so they suggested an alternative that would work in the confined space I had in the navigation station. I ended up buying a Mini-Mac which they configured to operate Windows XP, an elegant solution, I thought.

On July 5 our friends Stephen and Katie arrived. We spent the first evening getting them situated and making our final plans for Glacier Bay. We still didn't have a reservation, but we were hopeful it would come through. We would call at least three times a day from here on out, starting at 6:00 a.m., when they accepted the first reservation requests for the day, to hopefully secure a permit.

When we shoved off the next morning the skies were overcast and threatening rain, but we had good winds, so we managed to sail the 15 miles to the Lynn Canal. I had picked out a couple of likely anchorages that put us within an easy half-day sail of Glacier Bay, so if reservations could finally be confirmed, we'd be able to proceed there quickly. As we proceeded south through the Lynn Canal, the winds built to an uncomfortable 30 knots and we decided to put in at the first available port. A quick look at the chart revealed that Funter Bay was within six miles of our position, so we sailed into a small cove and dropped anchor for the night. In the morning, Sharon immediately used the satellite phone to check on our reservations and after several attempts we were granted a one-day reservation. We didn't have any idea how we could possibly see much of anything in the vast expanses of Glacier Bay in one day, but to borrow a strategy from the military, I thought if we established a 'beachhead,' things would probably sort themselves out.

We awoke to sunny skies and as soon as we entered Icy Strait we were treated to a grand show put on by several pods of humpback whales. We were delighted to observe behavior we hadn't seen before – repeated fin and tail slapping, as well as the more familiar breaching. As we approached the entrance to Glacier Bay, we encountered a significant number of sea otters sleeping on the surface. There was an 11:00 a.m. briefing at the Bartlett Cove Ranger Station and because the next one wasn't until 3:00 p.m. we really had to hit the throttle to make it in time for the morning session. It was a race and I was out of breath as I burst into the briefing room, but I'd just made it. The rest of the crew followed after securing the boat at the dock.

The ranger station was abuzz with activity. They were dealing with two separate emergencies. We were aware of both of them because we'd been monitoring their traffic on the VHF radio for several hours while *en route* from Funter Bay.

In the first instance, a sailboat was making an emergency stop at the ranger station to air evacuate an injured passenger. It didn't sound life-threatening, but serious enough to require that a plane be dispatched from Juneau to nearby Gustavus, from where they could transport the injured crew back to the hospital.

The second incident was potentially much more serious. A large cruise ship had run aground in Tarr Inlet on the falling tide and the ship was teetering high and dry on a large sandbar. One of the rangers commented that these were the situations they trained for, but that to have two at once was really taxing their resources.

Once things settled down a little, the briefing began. I had already picked out several anchorages I knew we wanted to try, so I took advantage of the opportunity to inquire about them. The first choice was a spot in Tarr Inlet, adjacent to the Margerie Glacier, suggested by a local tour boat operator we'd met in Auke Bay. We were interested to learn that this area had just reopened after a 20-year closure, due to bear activity. Whenever they have incidents between humans and bears, they send a team to camp at the location. If the bears continue to create problems, they close the area for a generation of bears. They told us they currently had a team at another location because there had been an incident two days earlier. As implausible as it sounds, they instructed all of us that if we had food and a bear came for it, we were not to give it up. In the area they were currently studying, a camper had been charged while eating some beef jerky. When we asked what happened to him, they said "Nothing, he passed out and the bear settled for absconding with the beef jerky." From the briefing, we proceeded directly to the gift shop, where they sold a form of pepper spray designed specifically to repel bears.

The rules grew more perplexing. We were given a permit valid only until midnight. Clearly, we weren't leaving then, although it would still only be dusk. The rules stated that we could anchor only in a place called Blue Mouse Cove, where we could stay pending issuance of a new permit, provided we did not pull the anchor off the bottom. We would be allowed to kayak and dingy around, and since the anchorage was adjacent to the Hugh Miller Inlet, there should be good places to explore.

The entire entrance to Glacier Bay is a whale-protection area where humpbacks feed, and since they usually feed close to shore, all vessels are required to remain at least a half-mile from land. These rules were strictly enforced and we heard one boat receive a warning for cutting a corner as they were leaving Bartlett Cove. Since we were free to roam around until midnight, we took a circuitous route to Blue Mouse Cove, visiting a seal rookery and a nesting area for several species of birds on the Marble Islands. It was a raucous place, and from time to time marauding eagles would invade the nesting grounds, causing havoc and a cacophony of agitated birds.

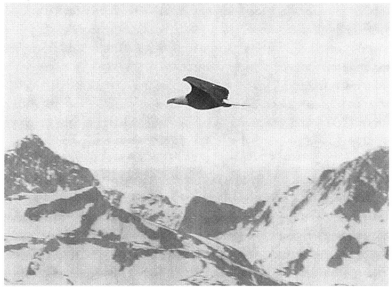

Nothing compares to the majesty of a bald eagle in flight.

Glacier Bay is a huge place. We sailed 35 miles from the Ranger Station in Bartlett Cove until we reached Blue Mouse Cove and we still had another 25 miles to go to our first glacier. Blue Mouse Cove reminded me of a detention camp. It turned out to be nondescript and bleak. I chuckled to myself as I was reminded of the detention I'd served a time or two in junior high school for misbehaving. There was an unoccupied ranger station tucked into one corner and we'd been told it was frequently manned, so we could have a watchful eye on us at any time. It was also a very difficult place to get the anchor to set. For the most part, we'd found the holding at all of the anchorages along our route to be excellent and our Manson state-of-the-art anchor more than capable. Here, however, we tried several times to set the anchor near a small creek outlet and finally had to cross the cove to find good holding ground. It was early evening by the time we arrived, and since we were all worn out from the day's events, we made an early night of it.

The day started out with bad news. Sharon was the first one up and called the rangers at 6:30 a.m., only to be told that no extension to our permit was available. It looked like we would be stuck in this ho-hum anchorage with not much to look at for another day. Deciding to make the most of it, we launched the dinghy and both kayaks, which I playfully referred to as my "fleet," and spent the next several hours exploring along the shore, taking short hikes and poking around for shells at a spot across the cove near where we'd first tried to anchor. When we returned to the boat for lunch around 2:00 p.m., on a hunch I decided to call Bartlett Cove to check our status, and lo and behold, they granted us a three-day extension on our permit. We dropped everything and immediately set sail for Tarr Inlet, opting to eat underway. This was the location of the cruise ship grounding, but we were beyond radio range of Bartlett Cove and wouldn't find out until much later that all the passengers were safely removed, and after a thorough survey by the ship's agents and the Coast Guard, it was safely re-floated and returned to Juneau for repairs. We missed the drama of that big event.

Tarr Inlet is home to Grand Pacific Glacier and Margerie Glacier, the most spectacular and active of them all. When we arrived at the upper reaches of Tarr Inlet, we were at the northernmost point of our journey, 59° north latitude. We'd almost reached the 60th parallel. This was the Holy Grail of our voyage and the first goal we had set for ourselves two years before. We didn't have time to dwell on our achievement, because the sights and sounds of the glacier a mere quarter-mile from our position were awe-inspiring. Margerie Glacier was very active and calved several times with a resounding crack as mountainsides of ice broke away and crashed to the waiting ocean below. One of these was a massive section from the center of the mile-long glacier which created a huge wave we thought was going to engulf us, but which fortunately dissipated to a manageable size on its march across the deep, ice-filled water.

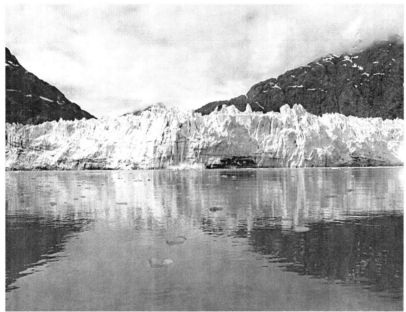

Margerie Glacier is the star of Glacier Bay.

After watching for almost an hour, it was time to head to our anchorage. It was only a mile from the glacier and we could enjoy the sights and sounds from this location as well. The entire upper end of Tarr Inlet was filled with icebergs and bergy bits which were almost too thick to pass as we approached the base of the glacier. Our anchorage was chock-full of bergy bits, but they were moving so slowly they didn't seem to present any danger. While the crew ate dinner, I kept a weary eye on the ice, occasionally using the fully extended boat hook to fend off some of the larger pieces. I didn't want the boat to get scratched, because many of these glacial remnants carried dirt and sharp rocks that weren't a serious threat, but could mar our otherwise near-pristine hull. What we hadn't anticipated was the effect of the changing tides. When the ebb started and huge quantities of the sea began to flow out of Tarr Inlet, it carried with it many of the larger icebergs we'd seen at the base of Margerie Glacier. It soon became clear that we'd be required to stand an overnight anchor watch. These larger icebergs had the capability of dislodging our anchor, setting us adrift in the dark of night in these treacherous waters. I agreed to stand the first watch, being a night owl anyway. I stayed up until 4:00 a.m. when Sharon took the second watch. Everyone else would be up by 7:00 a.m. or 8:00 a.m. to relieve her and I was planning to sleep late. When I finally awoke, I learned that Sharon had to awaken Stephen at 6:30 a.m. because a Volkswagen-sized iceberg was taking aim at us and she was afraid she didn't have the strength to fend it off. Stephen and I both commented that never in our wildest imagination had we envisioned ourselves fending off icebergs while at anchor.

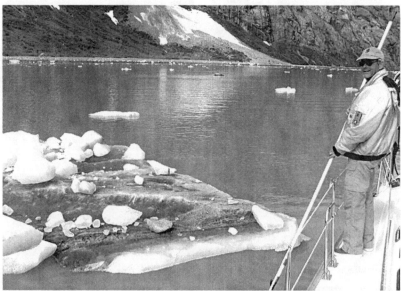

Sharon had to enlist Stephen's "muscle" to fend of this approaching iceberg.

Before lunch we all piled in the dinghy and headed back to Margerie Glacier. We decided to tow the kayaks, but it didn't work out too well because they filled with water, drenching the seats, so we all stayed in the dinghy. It was one thing to ride out a swell cre-

252

ated by calving ice in the relative safety of *Last Resort*, but quite another from the vantage point of our small dinghy. The glacier was even more active this day and there was a constant roar, creating thunderous echoes in the small inlet, as we all craned our necks to see where the latest ice had broken free. It wasn't long before we were joined by two large powerboats and a massive cruise liner. We felt minuscule as we lay trapped between the ice and the cruise ship holding station just beyond our vantage point. We sat motionless when a fishing boat unexpectedly appeared, and barely slowing, charged through the thick ice to the very base of the glacier. They had arrived so suddenly they couldn't have realized how active the glacier had been. Before long a sizeable section of ice calved dangerously close to them and they made a hasty retreat the way they'd arrived. Katie could have stayed all day, but after about an hour I started worrying about our boat, which we'd left unattended. After carefully working our way through the thick ice, even having to row at one point to protect the prop, we were back aboard and the crew settled down for lunch as I made preparations to weigh anchor.

Our next stop was Reid Glacier. As we departed our anchorage, the ice was so thick that I sent Sharon to the bow, wearing one of our hands-free headsets so she could direct me around the ice. She would assume this duty on numerous occasions during our stay in Glacier Bay. Reid Glacier itself wasn't nearly as majestic as Margerie Glacier because it was rapidly receding and was no longer considered a marine glacier. A large strip of exposed beach now separated it from the ocean waters. We decided to take the dinghy and the kayaks ashore. Stephen and Katie were going to do some hiking and Sharon and I planned to kayak to the base of the glacier and land on the beach. Shortly after we dropped Stephen and Katie off and securely tied the beached dinghy to a rock ashore, Sharon and I set out in the kayaks. We were in for a dangerous surprise. We'd heard plenty about williwaws.

Far from the safety of the shore, we were suddenly blasted with the frigid, 30-knot winds of a williwaw, the first we'd encountered. We immediately found ourselves straining to hold position in our kayaks, but as frantically as we peddled and paddled, we were rapidly losing ground. The risk was that we could have been blown completely out of the cove and left unable to get back. If *Last Resort's* anchor dragged in the heavy winds or Stephen couldn't get the dinghy outboard started, we could all be in real trouble. I'd given him a handheld VHF radio, but he either hadn't turned it on or couldn't hear me desperately trying to raise him. Finally, giving up all chance of returning to the dinghy, I signaled to Sharon that we should stop fighting and set a downwind course so we could angle toward the shore. We landed about a quarter-mile from the dinghy and found ourselves in sticky mud that made walking almost impossible. After what seemed like an eternity, I saw Stephen finally launching the dinghy to rescue us. It had been a close call and it took its toll on Sharon, whose usually chipper disposition had all but disappeared by the time we finally clambered back aboard *Last Resort*. Fortunately the anchor had held against the onslaught of the williwaw, which finally blew itself out after a few hours. Once the winds died, I didn't see the need to maintain an overnight anchor watch for the second night in a row, much to the approval of our crew. I stayed up late and was treated to the most spectacular sunset I can recall, the setting sun reflected in an orange blaze from the snow-covered peaks and the clouds hovering nearby, blurring any distinction between the two. The time was just before midnight.

The next morning we were greeted by the best weather we would experience during our entire summer in Alaska. The crew was awake early, while I chose to sleep in. When I finally came on deck, I found them sunning themselves in shorts and tee shirts. It was quite a sight to photograph Katie and Sharon dressed for tropical weather with Reid Glacier as the backdrop. The contradiction was remarkable.

The next day, our last, we'd planned an aggressive 60-mile route that would take us to another section of the park that promised views of still more spectacular glaciers. When we arrived at the McBride Glacier, we found the cove choked with icebergs the size of houses and we marveled at the bright blue of all the ice. It was stunningly beautiful. We debated launching the dinghy and trying to get closer, but the icebergs were packed tight and the risk seemed high. There was also an ominous looking weather front approaching from the north, so we decided we'd best head for Sandy Cove, the anchorage we'd settled on for the night. We had a cold ride in heavy rain and fog that reduced our visibility enough that we had to navigate using our radar. By the time we got there, Sandy Cove was already crowded, as a number of boats had come in earlier to avoid the storm. We finally found a small spot to drop our anchor and retired to the warmth of our cozy cabin. We couldn't stop talking about our adventures as we planned an early morning departure.

We could have stayed one more day in Glacier Bay, but the weather was foul and we elected to break up the return trip into two legs. A wise woman once told me, "Always leave while you're still having fun." We anchored about half-way back to Auke Bay in a scenic little spot called Swanson Harbor after a brisk sail back down Icy Strait. A day later we were back in Auke Bay and enjoyed our last night aboard with Katie and Stephen as they organized and packed for their early morning flight back to California.

Three days later there was another crew change. Sharon had to make a business trip to Florida and our friend Stephanie had agreed to fly up from Half Moon Bay to crew for me so I wouldn't be stuck in Auke Bay for a week with no company and nothing to do. I'd settled in advance on Port Frederick as a likely place to go exploring during Stephanie's short visit. We were not disappointed as we passed the unique rock formations and islets that dotted the southern end of this 15-mile bay. We anchored in Neeks Bay and enjoyed exploring the scenic shoreline by kayak. I was thrilled when the crab pot yielded my biggest catch yet, six crabs, four of which were large males, providing a feast for Stephanie. Our second night we stopped in the town of Hoonah, a prosperous First Nation hamlet. We had a good laugh at one of the notices tacked to the local bulletin board:

"Hooptie For Sale. Chevy pickup: If you've ever had a Chevy this has everything wrong that can go wrong. Plus a bonus: Blown Motor. If you're handy or enjoy walking, this beauty can be yours for $1000.00. It is the green pickup you

never see around town. Currently anchored in the front tri-
plex on Salmon loop. Good luck, or buy a Ford!"

When Sharon returned from Florida we had another day
together before Stephanie had to leave, so we set off to explore
Juneau. For the first time we wandered into the tourist area and
stopped for lunch at the Red Dog Bar, a *must* for the tourists visiting
Juneau aboard the cruise ships. After lunch, we had a fascinating
tour of the Alaska-Gastineau gold mine and paid one final visit to
the Mendenhall Glacier before heading back to the boat.

That night we engaged Stephanie, a public relations professional
like Sharon, in a conversation about the Sail Through Cancer Foundation. I hadn't had a lot of time to think about it since leaving San
Francisco, much less take any action. Stephanie asked me if I'd
reserved the domain name, and when I sheepishly admitted to not
even checking its availability, she sternly admonished me that I
needed to at least do that much.

Stephanie's flight was at 4:00 a.m., so it was a short night,
although Sharon and I went back to bed after seeing her off. We
had another day or two in Juneau, and heeding Stephanie's advice,
I was able to secure the domain name and started putting together
a temporary website for the to-be-formed foundation. As for us, it
was time to leave as well. *Last Resort* had overstayed her welcome
in Auke Bay and with August, which they call "Fogaust" in these
waters, only a few days off, we made good our escape, beginning
the return voyage to southern British Columbia with very mixed
emotions. We had 1200 miles to go and the promise of some
summer weather as we returned to lower latitudes.

Hoonah was a convenient stop, and since Sharon hadn't seen it,
we put in there our first night. The weather was dreadful and we
only left the boat for a short walk the following morning to take
some pictures. We were heading back, but our Alaskan adventures
were far from over. We'd decided to make the return voyage on the
"outside." I always felt confined by the channels of the Inside Passage and I wanted to experience sailing in the Gulf of Alaska. This
day proved to be the most enthralling sailing of the entire Alaskan
adventure. We set off for the 25-mile run down Icy Strait in 25-to-
30-knot winds that were dead astern. Almost immediately, I set the

whisker pole and wing-on-wing we sailed towards Elfin Cove, an eclectic hamlet tucked behind several sheltering islands along the western edge of the Gulf of Alaska. As we approached Point Adolphus we were treated to four different pods of humpbacks feeding all around us. Our silent approach, without the noise of the usually-throbbing engine, allowed us to pass peacefully between them, pushing the quarter-mile legal distance requirement to its limits. We marveled as they breached and cavorted. Some were even bubble feeding off in the distance. Bubble feeding is when the whales create a curtain of bubbles and slowly herd their prey into a small area where they can then breach, taking in massive amounts of food as they break the surface.

The serenity of these peaceful behemoths was soon to be brutally interrupted. As we entered the very narrow South Inian Pass before rounding the last headland between us and Elfin Cove, we noticed a large commotion in the waters dead ahead. As we approached, we couldn't immediately discern what was causing the ruckus, but we soon spotted a pod of Orcas and several humpbacks. In spite of the excitement of our Glacier Bay experience, the real drama of the trip was unfolding before our eyes, as we realized the Orcas were actually attacking a humpback calf. This was both tragic and compelling to watch. We could see the sow frantically flailing about and her plaintive cries were haunting and heart-rending. We did not stay to see the end and learn if the calf survived, although the outcome appeared inevitable.

When we entered Cross Sound rounding Point Lavinia, we had our first taste of open ocean in a long time. It felt good to see the expanse of the ocean again, with the horizon far, far off in the distance. When we arrived in Elfin Cove there was no room at the public float, but some very nice people on a beautiful 47-foot Grand Banks trawler offered to let us raft up next to them. I was still a little shaken from our approach to the docks, because as we entered the tiny cove a daredevil bush pilot decided he'd beat us in, and unaware of his approach, I nearly jumped overboard when he landed literally a few feet off our starboard side. I took a minute to compose myself before attempting the tricky docking maneuver alongside this beautiful yacht in the extremely tight quarters. Once securely tied off we were invited aboard for a drink. These people were from Portland, Oregon, and we exchanged contact information so that we might visit them on our way south, after we finally leave the Pacific Northwest.

Elfin Cove is a whimsical theater set behind fog's ethereal scrim. Bewitched, we tromped through a little hamlet apparently designed by elves at their most impish. It's an understatement that the people of Alaska are eclectic. Every one of the tiny hamlets we visited was peppered with random works of art, ranging from the huge spider web, complete with wrought iron spider, in Meyers Chuck, to a fanciful carving we found here, an abstract eel adorned with salmon berries. As Sharon bent to pose for a picture, the analogy to *Beauty and the Beast* was inescapable. The town was built on planks interlaced with ever-meandering boardwalks, the whole of which was suspended above the perennial damp of the Alaskan rain forest.

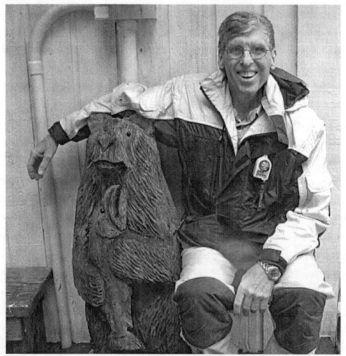

Elves have been busy carving eclectic art in Elfin Cove.

We would linger another day to explore every nook of this wonderland. The inner harbor was far too small to accommodate a vessel our size, but we wandered in by dinghy, exploring the far reaches of the cove and the cascading waterfall that fed fresh water, creating a brackish brew that accelerated the decay of several abandoned wrecks littering the shoreline. Amazingly, we saw very few souls in this tiny outpost that clawed its very existence from the rugged shore of the Gulf of Alaska.

However, we had one more "inside passage" before reaching the Gulf of Alaska, because we wanted to visit Pelican, another fabled hamlet with a boardwalk instead of sidewalks or streets. Visiting Rosie's bar, we no sooner slid onto a couple of bar stools than we met Rosie herself, a hardy, enterprising woman who's operated this self-proclaimed "World Famous" bar for over 30 years. We sat next to a fisherman who looked like the comedian Steven Wright (well-known for his unique observations, "Why do we drive on a parkway and park in a driveway?") and who spoke in the same soft mutter, causing us to strain to hear as we talked. "I left here yesterday, about this time," he remarks, engaging us easily in conversation (extraordinary for an Alaskan, actually). "I ran smack-dab into a grizzly out on the boardwalk!" He inserts a dramatic pause, noting our widening eyes. "I ran right back to Rosie's!" After visiting the other bar in town and looking around, we furtively headed back aboard for the night, on the lookout all the way.

Finally heading for open ocean, we sailed down the Lisianski Channel where a wonderful thing happened. The rain stopped, the sun shone and the breeze blew. Hoisting the sails and cranking up the volume on the stereo, we danced and sang. We would soon be free of the narrow confines and enjoying sunsets unimpeded by snow-covered mountains or green hills covered with pines. As we entered the Gulf of Alaska we had one last, humbling view of the ice-laden mountains we were leaving behind, maybe, probably, forever.

We were looking forward to visiting White Sulfur Hot Springs. The thought of soaking in a wilderness hot tub had real appeal after enduring so many bone-chilling days since arriving in Alaska.

259

We anchored in Porcupine Bay, a well-protected, cheerful spot with a view of the ocean and a torrential waterfall nearby. There is an anchorage much closer to White Sulfur Hot Springs, but one hair-pin turn in the channel entrance precluded a vessel our size from availing ourselves of the convenience. We were soon bouncing along over wind-driven chop as we sped towards Bertha Bay in the dinghy. Our reward was a long, luxurious soak in a black-granite, natural hot spring, over which the Forest Service had erected a small building, complete with a picture-window view of the bay and open ventilation allowing us to breathe in the refreshing salt air as we warmed ourselves in the hot mineral waters. By the time we got back, the sun was shining brightly and it had warmed up so much that I actually took a shower on the stern ladder, the first time I'd ever used the outdoor shower. I've had to remind some of my twittering friends of the complete solitude we experienced on this outside route, which very few cruisers ever experience. We lin-gered in the cockpit for hours and at sunset I was treated to a sky like I'd never seen before. In the movie *Voyage to the Bottom of the Sea*, the plot revolved around the atmosphere somehow catching fire. They didn't need any special effects for the movie, for had they only known, they could have come to Alaska and simply filmed what I was witnessing.

A large chunk of the Alaskan panhandle is consumed by three major islands, commonly referred to as the "ABCs," Admiralty, Baranof and Chichigof. The next day we were headed to Chichigof, a once-thriving mining town from which the island derives its name. But to get there, we first had to navigate "The Gate," the for-midable entrance to Klag Bay. Known for treacherous currents, at its worst The Gate has a depth of only 25 feet and a width of 50 yards. Our near-48-foot boat draws eight feet. A new friend we sub-sequently met in Ketchikan, who headed the Coast Guard Auxiliary there, told us that the Coast Guard estimates there are more than 104,000 uncharted rocks in southeastern Alaska, alone. (If they were counting them, why didn't they chart them, one won-dered?) We hoped there weren't too many on our way into Klag Bay. We white-knuckled it on the way through, carefully conform-ing to thoughtfully-placed range-markers, keeping one eye on the depth and the other on the chart-plotter. We did not time this passage at exactly slack tide, but our powerful engine pushed us through the outflow without difficulty. Once well inside Klag Bay, our eyes feasted on an inland archipelago with seemingly hundreds of tiny islets, coves and secluded anchorages. We opted to continue all the way to Chichigof at the head of the bay where we safely dropped anchor just a few yards offshore from the dilapidated ghost-town.

That night we spotted a shallow cove teaming with salmon. We knew they wouldn't be biting at this stage in their life cycle, but we thought if we dragged a three-pronged hook with a shiny lure we might get lucky and snag one. That didn't work out, but we enjoyed the ride and the scenery. Content, we returned to the boat.

Our good weather was giving way to a gray overcast so we decided to explore the ruins immediately, rather than wait until morning when it might well be raining. As we packed the camera and a few other things, I completely forgot to include the bear repellant we'd purchased in Glacier Bay. We were poking around the littered ruins and as I inspected a rusted old fuel tank, we were startled by the growls of two bears that had silently approached and were way too close for comfort. They say you're not supposed to run, but stand your ground when confronted by a bear. The thought of standing my ground never occurred to me, and apparently not to Sharon either, as we both instinctively sprinted the 25 yards to the dinghy, diving in head first and propelling it off the rocky beach. My hands were trembling as I fumbled to lower the outboard and get it started. Only then did we look back, relieved that we hadn't been pursued by these black bears, the kind we'd been told would have liked to have eaten us for supper.

We were headed for Sitka, but to break up the long voyage, I studied all the possible anchorages along the route and settled on Sukoi Inlet. It was three miles into the inlet to reach good anchorage and three miles out, but the weather was deteriorating rapidly and I thought we would appreciate the security of this well-sheltered alternative. As visibility dropped and the intensity of the rain increased we opted to bypass Sukoi Inlet when we reached that point. We had a good boost from the current and with favorable winds we were sailing at over seven knots, so we decided to continue on to Sitka, three hours beyond. We successfully navigated Neva Strait, mindful of the numerous rocks awash and shoals that must be avoided. Arriving in Sitka early in the evening, the only space was on the outer transient dock which lacked electrical hookups. We went on a waiting list, but it would be two days before we were accommodated in a slip. This marina uses what they call "hot berthing," or assigning transient boats to slips temporarily vacated by their permanent tenants, usually fishing boats heading out for periods of several days to a week or more.

We had a short respite of good weather once they moved us into a proper slip. Sharon suggested we take advantage of it and launch the kayaks so we could explore the Sitka waterfront. We were delighted when we rounded one corner to see a familiar boat in front of us and broad smiles spread on our faces as we read the name, "Un-Doc'd." Bucky and Christy were here, the name of their small trawler an apparent celebration of Bucky's retirement from the practice of medicine. Christy was an absolute hoot. I remember one night in Ketchikan, as she was describing some of the characters she'd encountered in Alaska, when she went on to say in her deep Alabama accent that "Everyone in this state looks like they're in the Witness Protection Program." We laughed out loud at that, because we'd met a number of people who, if not running from the law, were surely running from something. These friends had decided to leave their boat in Sitka and were winterizing it in preparation to haul it out for dry storage. We'd often commented that we should have become Hobie dealers, because everyone who saw our peddle-and-paddle kayaks wanted one. Bucky and Christy were no different and after they tried ours out, decided right on the spot to order two similar ones upon their return to Birmingham.

We spent a full week in Sitka, lingering to visit as long as we could before Christy and Bucky took off. Unable to find a mechanic who wasn't booked up solid with business from the fishing fleet, I managed to buy some oil and perform an oil change myself, as well as attend to other ship's chores. There was always something. This would be the last chance for awhile to obtain parts and we would soon be off-the-beaten-path. Sharon provisioned more fully than usual because we were heading to a sparsely-populated portion of southeast Alaska with few services. Other than a few fishermen, we didn't expect to see any other boats, but I was intrigued by descriptions I'd read of some of the anchorages and was in search of solitude. As soon as the latest shipment of mail arrived, we cast off our lines and made the very short sail to nearby Goddard Hot Springs. We'd enjoyed our first experience at White Sulfur Hot Springs so much that we'd researched at least two more which we planned to visit on the way back south. Goddard Hot Springs was a good choice, but we didn't have it to ourselves. There were two sets of tubs and the lower set next to the landing was occupied when we first arrived, so we hiked up the hill and enjoyed the panoramic views from the upper tub.

The next day turned out to be beautiful. The departure from Kliuocheovi Bay was exciting, as it was low tide and we saw a minimum of 9 feet under the keel as we maneuvered around several rocks that encumber the narrow channel entrance. We had planned a long passage that took us to an unnamed cove in the head of Puffin Bay on the southwestern tip of Baranof Island. We anchored in an exquisite basin, surrounded on all sides by mountains that rose to more than 2000 feet from our tiny sanctuary, lush green mountains with patches of snow that glistened in the rare sunshine we enjoyed that afternoon. I counted this location among my favorites, but my sentiments were not shared by the XO, who was ill-at-ease due to the preponderance of huge white jellyfish that densely populated the surrounding water.

Coronation Island was conveniently located along our route of travel from Baranof Island to Craig, another small Alaskan refuge. It reminded me of sailing to Catalina. We encountered flocks of puffins playfully bobbing on the water as we entered the anchorage, not far from a beautiful sand beach in a protected corner of the bay. As the anchorages were now serving up a menu of visual delights, we were making more use of our new kayaks and really getting our money's worth. We peddled and paddled along a rocky shore with lots of little inlets and big rocks totally surrounded by water, a gunkholer's delight. I remember one cylindrical rock tower that protruded in isolation and housed what looked to be a com-

263

plete ecosystem of plant life, much different from the surroundings. It was a wonderful outing. Sharon left her kayak in the water overnight so she could enjoy an early morning tour of another part of the bay we hadn't yet explored before our scheduled departure.

Our next stop was in Steamboat Bay, site of a long-since abandoned cannery. While we were in Elfin Cove, we'd learned why so many of the remote canneries had fallen on hard times. Our first night in Elfin Cove the fishing fleet had arrived. What drew them was a very large boat that had facilities to keep a huge amount of crab stored in circulating sea water and salmon in holds packed with beds of ice. These ships paid cash on the spot and had the ability to deliver huge quantities of seafood to market while still fresh. Confronted with this competition and the overall decline of the Alaskan fisheries in general, these small, isolated canneries simply couldn't compete.

Before we left San Francisco, we'd learned that the entire salmon fishery in California had collapsed, an environmental catastrophe, the far-reaching effects of which are still unknown. California acted quickly to close the upcoming salmon season, driving large numbers of fishermen into financial blight. Oregon and Washington would soon follow. Alaska, to the best of our knowledge, never completely closed the season, although we heard they had placed severe restrictions on the catch limits and the fisherman complained of the poor catches in all but a few areas. One fisherman we talked to in Sitka, who generously gave us several huge salmon-sections, since I'd had little time for fishing myself, blamed the dramatic declines on gill-netting by the Japanese and Chinese fishing fleets taking place farther out to sea. Our oceans, like much of the environment, are in need of preservation as well.

We lingered in Craig, another small town along our route, long enough to retrieve a shipment of mail and sit out a gale. It was getting late in the season by now and it looked like we'd be among the last recreational boats to leave Alaska before winter set in. We had Internet service in Craig, and since we were closed-in by the storm raging outside, I used the opportunity to work on the Foundation website and to start researching the information I needed to incorporate and obtain the necessary 501(c)(3) tax exemption from the

Internal Revenue Service. Stephanie, it seemed, had really lit a fire under me, for I was also able to recruit a Board of Directors composed of luminaries from the medical and business world. I also started recruiting individual skippers to volunteer for the Armada of Hope, my name for the fleet of boats I planned to assemble to take cancer survivors and their loved ones out for a boat ride. It is the Foundation's premise that even a brief break from the rigors of cancer treatment and recovery can have a profound effect on those afflicted, particularly children, their families, caregivers and community of friends and associates.

After four days we finally got a break in the weather and headed out to a place called Clam Cove. It was on this leg that we had our first real problem with currents. Our route of travel took us through Tlevak Narrows. I'd checked the currents on the Raymarine chartplotter and was sure our arrival at the northern entrance was well-timed to coincide with slack tide. Preoccupied with my work on the Foundation, I didn't take the time I might otherwise have to double check the data against the Maptech charts on the ship's computer. As we approached Tlevak Narrows, my greatest navigation challenge lay just around the next point. Entering the north entrance to Tlevak Narrows something was terribly wrong. The red entrance buoy was hardly visible as it strained at its moorings, barely holding station against the onrushing current of rapidly rising water. The water ahead was a boiling cauldron of dangerous eddies. Motioning Sharon to take the wheel, I bolted below and pulled up the tidal data on the computer. Much to my shock, we were heading into the full force of the spring ebb, with the outgoing current running near its maximum velocity. At full throttle, I can easily achieve our rated hull speed of approximately 8.6 knots, but here I was hampered by the need to avoid the swirling eddies, some of which looked big enough to swallow a boat even our size. As I was weaving and bobbing along an erratic course fit only for a drunkard, I watched in anguish as our actual speed over the ground measured by the GPS started dropping, seven knots, five knots, four knots, three knots, two knots. Would we be able to forge through or were we destined to lose complete control as the current fed us to the deep or dashed us against one of

265

the multitude of uncharted rocks that appeared where the chart showed nothing but safe, unobstructed water? For the next hour, I struggled as we inched through the two-mile-long narrows, clutching the wheel to maintain control as my hands cramped and my shoulders burned. We had entered the height of the ebb tide and the conflicting currents tossed our vessel about like a rowboat in a maelstrom. I don't remember Sharon uttering a single word as I battled for our survival, but the terrified look on her face said it all.

As we finally emerged victorious at the south end of Tlevak Narrows, I remembered a discussion thread I'd followed on the Catalina 470 Association message board bemoaning the inaccuracy of some of the tidal data that came bundled with the electronic charts. I'd noticed minor discrepancies before, but this was huge and could have cost us our boat and even our lives. We won't soon forget that passage. I'd learned my lesson and from here on all tidal and current data was cross-checked.

One thing about this trip, there was never time to dwell on one thing for long, and this incident was no different. When we arrived at our destination, we discovered that the shoreline dropped off suddenly, but since there was good holding, we were able to anchor just a few yards off the beach. It was low tide and we had quite a treat when we were greeted by a beach-combing black bear which wandered in and out of the adjacent forest for the better part of the next two hours. Again we had warm weather. This was only the fifth truly warm day we'd experienced since we first arrived in Alaska, and it would prove to be our last.

We motor-sailed the next day in misty, overcast weather with dense fog that reduced our visibility to what we could see on the radar and not much else. We activated our fog horn and listened as it sounded its electronically-generated warning every two minutes for the next 40 miles. It was a long trip, so Sharon and I took turns on watch, which worked out well because I preferred to maintain a radar watch from down below while Sharon was in the cockpit, although we hadn't seen another boat since leaving Craig and it was unlikely we would. We were headed for Gardner Bay, a desolate anchorage on Prince of Wales Island that looked protected and scenic from the chart and the descriptions in the sailing instructions. Like many of our anchorages, this one, too, was entered through a narrow gap between a small island and the shore. Just as we entered we were caught off guard as a whale surfaced and spouted center channel, dead ahead. I didn't know how it was going to pass us in the narrow, shallow channel and I hoped it wouldn't stave us out of defensive fear. It sounded quickly and safely avoided our keel as it inched by.

This cove was among the more scenic we'd visited and we couldn't wait to jump in the kayaks. We peddled and paddled almost a mile. First we visited an interesting little waterfall that was fed from a salt water lake that fills at high tide and then drains both salt and fresh water at low tide. The brim was at least 15 feet above sea level while we were there, so we calculated the tidal changes must easily exceed 20 feet at times. I made a mental note to double check the tide tables, as well as the depth and scope of the anchor and chain we'd deployed when we first arrived. After landing the kayaks among some sheltered rocks, we climbed to the brim to get a good look at this phenomenal feature.

From there, we paddled to a small inlet we'd first seen when entering Gardner Bay at high tide and which looked like we could enter in the kayaks. But now, at low tide, the inlet could only be navigated for a short distance before we ran out of water. That inlet had an intriguing shoreline and I got some great pictures of jelly-fish and starfish near the entrance

Before I headed for the shower, I turned on the generator to charge up the batteries. Our friends Clark and Nina had warned us once before about the large orange jellyfish, the Lions Mane that I'd noticed were thick in the water surrounding the boat. I paid little attention to these extremely dangerous jellyfish and their highly toxic tentacles, as I had no intention of getting anywhere near one, or so I thought. Shortly after turning on the generator, I noticed that the sound of sea water running through the exhaust suddenly stopped, so I quickly shut it down and began to investigate. What I found was that one of these gooey creatures had been sucked into the raw water intake and had completely clogged the intake and the sea water strainer. Even though I took precautions while clean-ing it out, I managed to sustain some nasty stings. In some pain and concerned it would get worse, I called the Coast Guard for advice. They told me to treat the wounds with vinegar, and absent that, to use urine, confirming what I thought was a joke when a bunch of local fisherman chimed in on the VHF suggesting just that remedy – in far more colorful language. When the vinegar didn't do much, I opted to follow another anonymous fisherman's unsolicited advice to "Just man up," rather than try the urine approach.

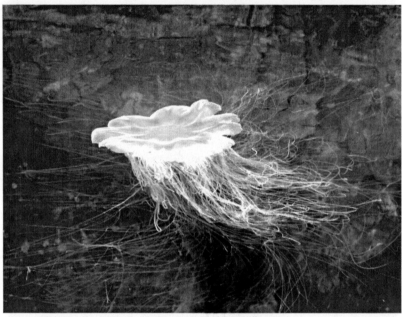

*Lions Mane jellyfish can deliver a **debilitating** sting.*

Throughout our Alaskan odyssey we were comforted by the diligent concern for our well-being that Darlene, assisted by her husband Floyd, repeatedly demonstrated as we made our daily check-ins with the Great Northern Boaters' Net. We had grown very fond of Darlene and were going out of our way to pay her a visit before we left Alaska forever. They lived on what can only be described as an outpost they'd manufactured with their bare hands on a small island so remote that it was beyond the reach of any local government. The handmade tree house reminded us of Tom Sawyer's Island in Disneyland. Darlene was adding shakes of cedar to the roof one at a time. Floyd and a buddy had arduously built the house on stilts by hand.

With statehood, Alaska started the job of taming its diverse territories and was slowly annexing them to the various Burroughs the legislature had established. Darlene and her small band of neighbors had steadfastly resisted and managed to retain their treasured autonomy, up until then, anyway.

Their next door neighbor had constructed a substantial dock, and since they'd already left for the winter, Darlene instructed us to tie up there, where we'd be secure for the night. As we rounded the corner into the tiny channel they called home, Darlene jumped in her skiff and led us to our landing. She visited for three hours. No wonder she runs a radio network, Darlene is a talker, and also a lovable character. Over dinner Floyd told us a chilling story. There was a resident pod of Orcas here in Dora Bay and only two weeks earlier, one of their neighbors and his wife had ventured out onto the bay for some halibut fishing. Having better luck than I'd ever experienced, they'd landed a 140-pound halibut. Before they could manhandle this beast into the skiff, one of the Orcas surfaced and wrested it from their clutches. To add insult to injury, the Orcas began circling their small boat and started bumping it in an effort to catapult them into the frigid waters. They aimed their tiny aluminum boat at full throttle for the nearest shore, while the woman maintained the presence of mind to videotape the remainder of the incident as the whole pod of Orcas gave chase. They never cut the throttle, electing to drive the dinghy far up the seaweed covered shore while the Orcas just lingered close astern as if to warn them they weren't going to stand mortal humans competing for their food. We saw that pod of Orcas as we departed the next morning and were glad to have our five feet of freeboard between us and them as they passed close aboard.

We'd scheduled a short stop in Ketchikan to retrieve the mail and attend to any last minute business or repairs before we headed back to British Columbia. The weather forecast was not good and we'd left over the protests of Darlene and Floyd who'd wanted us to stay longer. I was worried we'd be stuck for two or three days if the oncoming weather was as bad as was being forecast, and as we sailed across Clarence Strait, we got a small taste of the weather that was to come.

This time our preference was Bar Harbor at the northern end of Ketchikan. It was closer to a major grocery store and the marina office, where our mail would arrive. Thirty minutes out I radioed the marina to secure a slip. Much to my surprise another voice broke in on the conversation asking if we could be moored near them. We were overjoyed to discover that Lou and Mary were still in Ketchikan. We thought they'd be long gone by now, but mechanical issues had delayed them in Auke Bay and taking different routes, we'd once again arrived within hours of each other. It proved to be a blessing that they were there, because Alaska wasn't quite ready to release its hold on us. We sat in Ketchikan for 10 days as gale after gale lashed our rigging and made us all but prisoners on our own boat. We did meet some wonderful people while we were there and weather-be-damned, we had a party almost every night.

When we finally escaped we had planned to buddy boat to Prince Rupert with *Seventh Heaven* and make the entire passage in one run, as we'd done when we arrived. It was not to be, for Alaska took one final swipe in an attempt to keep us, and we were forced to seek refuge in Foggy Bay when the deteriorating conditions ruled out crossing Dixon Entrance.

We'd sailed *Last Resort* more than 3,000 miles in order to relish the experience of an Alaskan-sized jellyfish, having started in Ensenada, Mexico, beaten our way northward along the U.S. coast, meandered through Canada's Inside Passage, wandered – spellbound, starry-eyed, mouths agape – through Glacier Bay National Park and hop-scotched our way southward through a virtual minefield of rock-strewn coast. Countless hours of tedium punctuated by occasional life-threatening incidents had brought us through some sort of spiritual transition. Our fears had each been taken out and examined before being repackaged and stowed deeper in the hold. We'd achieved a heady disconnect from limits. So, thank you very much, Alaska. I dare say I'd learned to "Just man up!"

Epilogue

"You're going to die from something, but it won't be this neck and throat cancer." Those were the last words my oncologist said to me as he wished me *bon voyage* before we set sail on this journey. I've been blessed to have regained the health of my younger years, with the obvious exception of the pesky problem of not being able to eat, which has by now been relegated to the category of "annoyance," as opposed to some dire handicap. So what's in store for *Last Resort* as her voyages continue?

As I write this, the U.S. economy has experienced the worst meltdown of our lifetime, but the country is filled with optimism, as am I, since the inauguration of a new president, Barack Obama, and a hopeful change of direction. We plan to continue on with our original plans in spite of it all. Our next adventure will be in Mexico.

To make the long winter pass more quickly here in British Columbia, I've already purchased a cruising guide and electronic charts for Central America. We are dreaming of tropical palms swaying in warm breezes as we watch snow piling on our deck. British Columbia and the entire Pacific Northwest are having a record-breaking winter — just our luck. Come spring we look forward to spending our allotted time in the State of Washington, exploring Puget Sound and the San Juan Islands. We'll need to bid our farewells to this pristine cruising ground and the many friends we've made along the way by mid-August, lest we run the risk of being captive for another winter. That will give us over two and a half months to reach San Diego in time to join the southbound fleet in late-October. We plan to join the Baja Ha-Ha for the annual autumnal migration in the fall, 2009. We will sail much farther into Mexico this time and cross over the Sea of Cortez to the mainland.

After Central America, we'll pass through the Panama Canal and spend a long time in the Caribbean. My memories of the Caribbean are fond and rich, but I've only scratched the surface of this playground in paradise. There will be much to discover and new cultures to absorb as we travel from country to country, island to island. The planet, as we perceive it, will continue to shrink.

One of our daughters lives with her husband in Germany and is planning a family in the near future, so with the prospect of a grandchild on the other side of the "Pond," we'll likely sail to the Mediterranean sooner rather than later, and use the boat as a base from which to explore all of Europe. Sharon will be near her future grandchild, but independent enough not to be a pest. Croatia, Greece and Turkey hold a particular allure for us and we hope to visit them as well.

The successful implementation of the Sail Through Cancer Foundation's mission to help other cancer sufferers has given meaning and purpose to my life. It is my passion to see this endeavor succeed and I will be devoting many of my waking hours to its success.

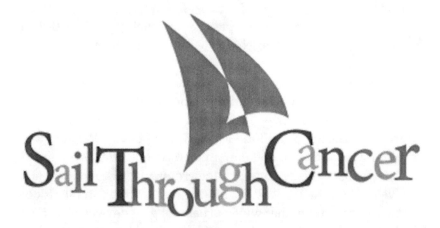

The fact that you're reading this means you probably enjoyed my story. I'm planning to have a lot more stories to tell, so who knows, perhaps you can look forward to a second book in the not too distant future.

Until then, fair winds!

Printed in the United States
142557LV00002B/4/P

9 780980 151213